The Bioethics of Enhancement

The Bioethics of Enhancement

Transhumanism, Disability, and Biopolitics

Melinda Hall

LEXINGTON BOOKS
Lanham • Boulder • New York • London

Published by Lexington Books
An imprint of The Rowman & Littlefield Publishing Group, Inc.
4501 Forbes Boulevard, Suite 200, Lanham, Maryland 20706
www.rowman.com

Unit A, Whitacre Mews, 26-34 Stannary Street, London SE11 4AB

Hall, Melinda. 2013. "Vile Sovereigns in Bioethical Debate." *Disability Studies Quarterly* 33, No. 4. Accessed July 31, 2016. doi: 0.18061/dsq.v33i4.3870.

Hall, Melinda. 2016. "Horrible Heroes: Liberating Alternative Visions of Disability in Horror." *Disability Studies Quarterly* 36, No. 1. Accessed July 31, 2016. doi: 10.18061/dsq.v36i1.3258.

Hall, Melinda. 2013. "Reconciling the disability critique and reproductive liberty: The case of negative genetic selection." *International Journal of Feminist Approaches to Bioethics* 6, No. 1: 121–143. Reprinted with permission from University of Toronto Press (www.utpjournals.com).

British Library Cataloguing in Publication Information Available

Library of Congress Cataloging-in-Publication Data
Names: Hall, Melinda Gann, author.
Title: The bioethics of enhancement : transhumanism, disability, and biopolitics / Melinda Hall.
Description: Lanham : Lexington Books, [2017] | Includes bibliographical references and index.
Identifiers: LCCN 2016043857 (print) | LCCN 2016044239 (ebook) | ISBN 9781498533485 (cloth : alk. paper) | ISBN 9781498533492 (Electronic)
Subjects: LCSH: Medical innovations—Moral and ethical aspects. | Medical innovations—Social aspects. | Medical innovations—Government policy. | Bioethics.
Classification: LCC RA418.5.M4 H35 2017 (print) | LCC RA418.5.M4 (ebook) | DDC 174.2—dc23
LC record available at https://lccn.loc.gov/2016043857

♾™ The paper used in this publication meets the minimum requirements of American National Standard for Information Sciences—Permanence of Paper for Printed Library Materials, ANSI/NISO Z39.48-1992.

Printed in the United States of America

Contents

Acknowledgments

I am forever grateful to my undergraduate professor, Lucinda Joy Peach. After my first class with her at American University, I declared Professor Peach harsh and unforgiving and vowed never to take another of her classes; yet, her name liberally peppers my transcript. When I graduated, after working with her on my senior capstone project, Lucinda gifted me a copy of *Prenatal Testing and Disability Rights* (ed. Parens and Asch), linking it with my interest in disability rights and ethics. Lucinda passed away that year, but her gift and memory have followed me as I pushed through graduate school, spent time at the Hastings Center learning from Erik Parens, and had the honor of briefly knowing the incredible Adrienne Asch. Lucinda's philosophical example, and that book, appear as a tight knot within the aim of the present work. I am further significantly indebted to Lucinda's example as a college professor; her voice and manner follow me in my own teaching as I attempt to carve out, as she did so capably for me and my classmates, a dynamic space for learning.

The research presented here was initiated at Vanderbilt University, where I completed my Ph.D. I am grateful to the University and Philosophy Department for generously providing the material support for conferences and research. For spiritual support, I must thank the brilliant individuals I had the tremendous fortune to study under and alongside and our many thousands of conversations, planned and incidental. I think especially of Rebecca and Garrett, without whom I would have lacked courage. Their friendship, energy, and incredible kindness in those years was just what I needed, and at just the right time, to grow and change. Kelly Oliver, my beloved dissertation supervisor and do-it-all mentor, is the light I follow personally and professionally. I admire her beyond measure. Kelly's leadership and "response-ability" brought me through graduate school to a career in academic philosophy. Without her, this book could not exist. Thanks are also due to Lisa Guenther, who provided me with detailed and invaluable comments on earlier drafts (the impact of which is sprinkled throughout these pages), and to Charles Scott, whose support and kindness kept me going at key moments in my project.

At Stetson University, I continued, refined, and deepened the research presented here, eventually bringing the project to completion. My thanks are due to the Dean's office and the Philosophy Department for their unflagging support of my research. I am also thankful for the friendship of my treasured colleagues and the significant ways they challenge me to consider the pursuit of philosophy anew. Our diverse voices together comprise a searching, at times surprising, but always valuable conversation. Thanks go to Joshua Rust in particular for our daily conversations. Thanks go also to my many fabulous students, especially those in my ethics classes, for considering with me the terrifically difficult problems represented by this book.

In the larger academic community, my thanks are due everywhere and are especially difficult to reckon. Many remarkable voices in philosophy and disability studies precede me and enrich my work. Shelley Tremain, in particular, encouraged me in my perspective, wonderfully setting out ways of thinking about disability through and with Michel Foucault in her incredible body of work. Conference attendees, panelists, commentators, and friends listened thoughtfully to my ideas and provided comments which shaped my research across several years at the American Philosophical Association, the Society for Phenomenology and Existential Philosophy, the Society for Disability Studies, and Western Michigan University's Ethics Center, as well as other organizations. My thanks are also due to an anonymous reviewer for Lexington Books whose feedback on my use of Foucault was enormously helpful. The work in this book has been reviewed in different venues by many other generous and accomplished scholars, to whom I am very grateful. Remaining errors are my responsibility.

Finally, my greatest thanks are due to my family. My mother, Linda, my first teacher and a fountain of encouragement, taught me to write (and diagram sentences). She has always been just a phone call away, an invaluable resource I abused many times. My father, Jon, subtly intimated to me at a very early age that philosophy was magic by shelving Nietzsche alongside Tolkien alongside theology in the study. My siblings, Andrea, Christina, and Justin, who are all so different, contributed in innumerable ways to whom I am today. I especially thank Christina for her incredible friendship, her joy at my successes, and her presence when things were hardest. Susan, Michael, and Ali, thank you for your strength, laughter, and constancy. For the incredible lightness of best friendship, love's buttresses and heights, and the perfect poached egg, I have Steven to thank. You bring me to life. And for our walks, well-timed naps, and important interruptions—thanks to my ridiculous and precious dog, who goes by many names.

Introduction

Enhancement, Disability, and Biopolitics

This book is based on a double contention. First, I claim that at the center of the debate over human enhancement is the question of disability—that is, a calling into question of disability, its value, and its meanings. Second, the debate over enhancement significantly shares questions and presuppositions concerning improving human life, happiness and its maximization, and enhancing human capacities with bioethics literature more generally. Debates in bioethics over analysis and communication, end-of-life issues, reproductive choice, rights, and justice, health resource allocation and rationing, the use of emerging technologies, and more are conditioned by assumptions about what makes life worth living and who should live. These assumptions, endemic in bioethics literature, are found in full bloom in literature promoting enhancement.

If disability underpins the enhancement debate, and the enhancement debate rests at the conceptual center of bioethics, disability—along with its value and meanings—is revealed as a major fulcrum for bioethics. Indeed, scholars in the philosophy of disability and disability studies have long drawn attention to the centrality of disability in bioethics. For instance, Tom Koch argues that bioethics shares a set of fundamental values and so is ideologically unified, and this ideology is hostile to disability. He identifies a "posture" in bioethics that is "agnostic, eugenic, and utilitarian" and which "denies the existential worth of any individual human being, and especially the individual of difference" (2006, 253; cf. Koch 2004). Writes Koch, "In contemporary bioethics the protected individual is protected only as long as he or she measures up in the sense that his or her social niche is acceptably cost efficient" (2006, 263). Meanwhile, Shelley Tremain connects bioethics tightly with politics and situates the discourse as a "predictable product and tangible outcome of" the movement of power in society, specifically in the mode of what Michel

Foucault articulates as *biopower* (2008, 101).[1] In the milieu of bioethics as biopower, Tremain argues that "differences [are] made perceptible as pathology, while the subjects who come to bear them are rendered as defective, are disabled, and signified as less than fully human" (102). Disability rights movements, eventually producing the field of disability studies and, more recently, the philosophy of disability, resisted and continue to resist these moves in bioethics, demonstrating Foucault's contention that power is always paired with resistance (102–103).

Bioethics is an academic and professional field in which experts are asked to establish protocols for and critically react to the role of medicine in everyday life, evolving technologies which mediate bodies and environments, and relationships between medical professionals and patients. Bioethics is, then, a network of relations in which power differentially operates. Understanding bioethics as a discourse of power means understanding it as a means to, for instance, judge who can speak, whose testimony counts, and what decisions are permissible in the clinical setting and at home. Many people are routinely excluded from speaking on their own behalf. Protocols surrounding informed consent provide some with the ability to consent to medical procedures and others with substituted judgment. Persons with disabilities provide testimony with regard to their quality of life but are deemed unreliable or deluded and their lives are considered not worth living (Goering 2008; Peace 2012, 2013b). This framework delimits and shapes the practice of medicine. Persons with disabilities experience significant health-care access issues, including the refusal of transplants (Buck 2016; Cohen 2013; Mitra *et al.* 2015). Women express their experiences of pain but are dismissed by their primary care physicians and go undiagnosed or misdiagnosed (Hoffman and Tarzian 2001; Munch 2004). Medical professionals act as gatekeepers for prescription drugs and regulate access to medical procedures. Desires among patients and laypersons to achieve increased autonomy, for example with regard to the time and manner of one's death, often serve only to further ensconce those in the medical profession as the primary means to that autonomy (Salem 1999). Yet, some are empowered through bioethics discourse and the practice of medicine. For instance, those with typical embodiment and spending power can expect access to medical care tailored to their needs and desires and the normalization of those needs and desires.

In short, bioethics is comprised of discourses and connects with medical practices which regulate whose voices, bodies, needs, and desires count. In bioethics literature, human subjects are drawn up against virtual ideals, especially against images of unfettered agency and rational choice. Echoing Tremain, I argue that bioethics is a medium of biopower insofar as it is a political organ, a normative discourse, and a gatekeeper. Given this, and given my contention that disability is hidden at the center of the enhancement debate, I approach bioethical debate over enhancement using a disability lens paired with Foucauldian analysis. I demonstrate that this framework yields major insights regarding who, how, and under what circumstances we are encouraged to consider enhancement obligatory or permissible.

To confront the enhancement debate head-on, I closely read the most enthusiastic proponents of human enhancement in the field of philosophy, *transhumanists*, and investigate their desired posthuman futures. Transhumanists pursue extended autonomy, multiplied choice, and enhanced moral acumen. Transhumanists dream of a future in which humans have transcended current capabilities in these areas through the use of emerging technologies aimed toward cognitive and physical augmentation. As I will show, these images of transcendence are desired escapes from embodiment, which is interpreted in this discourse as undesirable and risky vulnerability. Transhumanist bioethics mediates between the dream of the enhanced human—the posthuman—and the protocols, procedures, and discourses surrounding, inhibiting, and constituting the identities of those considered unfit for the future. In an amplification of the effects of bioethics more generally, transhumanism is tied up in the task of defining who counts and, therefore, who gets to live.

Considering disability in tandem with Foucault's work on biopower allows us to see, as I will argue, that enhancement enthusiasm in its contemporary iteration is not genuinely about enhancement at all. Current ideas in enhancement literature are focused on the level of the population, recommending enhancement for no one in particular, while particular individuals are deemed unworthy to live. The underlying question of enhancement enthusiasm, who should live, drives the debate over enhancement and should provoke anyone seriously committed to disability rights to object to the terms and assumptions of the discourse and rewrite the concept of enhancement. Currently enhancement discourse serves only to enhance our sense of risk and catastrophe, and enhances the conceptual linkage between disability and risk. Meanwhile, enhancement, in a variety of registers, is framed as inevitably a matter of bodily intervention. We should reconsider enhancement in terms of political and social intervention. This is particularly urgent given that the problems outlined in enhancement literature are political and social, yet the causes of these problems are reduced to biological factors.

For example, Ingmar Persson and Julian Savulescu contend there is an evolutionary explanation for what they claim is a universal tendency to focus on the good of those nearest us and ignore large-scale problems, to our existential peril (2012, 4). They, accordingly, suggest we must augment our moral progress through physical intervention like drug treatment and genetic engineering (107). Moral education and related development do not move quickly enough on their own to meet the catastrophes of climate change and terrorism (among other problems) (106).[2] Savulescu and Persson claim that human beings generally have a "parochial" or "common-sense" morality, inherited from an early pack or herd setting, and this parochial morality makes it difficult for us to be sympathetic to distant others. We are concerned about our own immediate "kin" and, as a result, we have difficulty reacting appropriately to large-scale problems of the sort that plague us today—that is, war, hunger, poverty, and climate change. Without serious moral adjustments—which these authors believe are possible via radical enhancement technologies—they worry we will never overcome the collective action problems that bar us from solving these issues. Savulescu and Persson argue that our moral ineptitude will cause us to become extinct if moral enhancement—specifically, effort to make humans more altruistic—is not undertaken (2012). In what follows, I will reject the turn to biology to solve political and social problems, the backdrop of risk and catastrophe that presents a false dilemma between certain disaster and enhancement, and the moral materialism evident in this account and those like it.

In these pages, I do not engage in the typical scuffles in the enhancement debate—such as defining the line between therapy and enhancement, or between cosmetic and reparative surgery. Instead, I pursue the question of enhancement directly by analyzing the work of strong advocates of the necessity for human enhancement. Prominent among these are philosophers Julian Savulescu and Nick Bostrom, who have global influence in bioethics. I am chiefly interested in the particular strategies these transhumanists suggest for enhancement and enhanced futures.[3] Further, I seek to reveal how they evaluate current circumstances and characterize existing persons as compared to the hoped-for posthuman. In short, I trace the material effects and points of view, applicable today rather than tomorrow, within Bostrom's and Savulescu's work in order to better morally assess their suggestions.

One may object that I skirt thorny issues in enhancement literature. Yet, introducing the centrality of disability to the issues surrounding enhancement, a centrality which is typically not treated in enhancement literature, changes the issues at hand significantly. Using the distinction between therapy and enhancement as a brief example can demonstrate this. This distinction disintegrates when we set aside the normativity of the abled body. To maintain the distinction between therapy and enhancement, one must endorse a norm such as Norman Daniels' species-typical functioning, which would set up a standard by which achievement of the norm would signify therapy and movement beyond the norm would signify enhancement (Daniels 1985). Refusing to endorse this concept or one like it opens the door to the question of why dismissing or denigrating the disabled body is central to enhancement debate. Further, transhumanists, the strongest proponents of enhancement, do not endorse the concept of the species-typical body as normative, as they find all current human bodies wanting and in need of improvement.

So, to the contrary, I do not skirt thorny issues; instead, I attempt to recalibrate and better engage the debate by bringing disability into sharp and sustained focus and largely avoiding distracting and hazy distinctions. I return to this issue in Chapter 1.

More importantly, one will ask why some quite helpful and nuanced scholars do not receive more attention and analysis here. For example, Nicholas Agar's excellent work on enhancement receives only brief mention. Why eschew the moderate Agar in favor of the work of provocateurs such as Bostrom and Savulescu? Indeed, one might contend, if I mean to seriously critique arguments for enhancement, I should consider the best and most careful arguments for enhancement, not the most enthusiastic. Scott Aiken and Robert Talisse explicate the problem at hand, christening it the "weak man fallacy," which they identify as a variant of the straw man fallacy (2014, 73). The weak man fallacy is at play when one seeks to critique a claim but chooses to refute a very weak argument for that claim, rather than available, better arguments. Using the straw man fallacy, one makes a viable argument sound worse than it is so that it is easy to critique. Using the weak man fallacy, one selects a bad argument from the beginning so that one can more easily succeed. Daniel Dennett treats this problem, too, in his recent popular book *Intuition Pumps* (2013). There, he lays out what he takes to be key rules for critical thought. For him, "there is a lot of mediocre work done in every field" and that a successful critical thinker should "go after the good stuff, or leave it alone" (2013, 36). He tells us to "make sure you concentrate on the best stuff you can find, the flagship examples extolled by leaders of the field, the prize-winning entries, not the dregs" (37). This seems reasonable and is attractive to anyone who pursues academic debate out of a love of wisdom.

Yet, its attractiveness aside, pursuing only the best arguments counts as a sound policy only if one assumes that the best arguments are the ones with the most influence in social and political registers. Unfortunately for us, the most influential and ideologically central arguments are not necessarily the best arguments. Assumptions made by Bostrom and Savulescu and those in their academic circles may be provocative—even specifically calibrated for a strong reaction—but they have strong purchase in literature on enhancement and both Bostrom and Savulescu are cited widely. Further, viewpoints expressed by Bostrom and Savulescu are shared in outline by laypeople as well as working and academic medical and genetics professionals. Consider the transplant board who refuses a new organ to a patient with a disability (Cohen 2013) or the genetics counselor who conflates genetic markers for Down syndrome with a fifty-percent chance of significantly impaired cognitive ability (Elkins and Brown 1995, 18 cited in Carlson 2002, 209; I return to this point in Chapter 4). This book is aimed toward social and political problems in everyday practical life, and what arguments matter in everyday life are very often not the best arguments. I seek instead arguments which rest at the rough knot among the threads of disability, risk, and enhancement. I hope to go some distance in untangling these concepts.

To this end, I ground and historicize the question of enhancement by turning my attention toward those found unfit at different moments throughout the twentieth century. Since the negative image of the utopian vision of the posthuman is always actually existing persons, I connect this negative image with those individuals thought to bear it—especially people with disabilities—and explore the ways that disability is constructed and stigmatized. I argue that transhumanists today do not offer a progressive politics of grander human diversity and autonomy, but rather a regressive politics—a politics of biological reduction and social exclusion. This politics pins social and political hope for the future, which they claim would otherwise be catastrophic, on the successful management, exclusion, and eventual elimination of risks discursively linked to disability.[4] Transhumanists desire maximized choice, but, in their pursuit of maximizing choice, actually eliminate choice for already-existing persons, thus closing off futures before they begin.[5]

With the aim of grounding and historicizing in view, I turn now to lay out Foucault's analysis of biopolitics and situate it as my theoretical frame and springboard for critiquing enhancement discourse. Michel Foucault was a French philosopher whose work impacted a wide variety of academic fields. To name just a few areas to which he significantly contributed, his work is used in gender studies, criminology, history, and psychology. From 1970 until his death in 1984, Foucault held a chair in "The History of Systems of Thought" at the Collège de France. In this position, he was required to hold public lectures each year. These are in the process of being published in their entirety. Many of Foucault's key concepts, like abnormality, security, subjectivity, the will to know, and biopolitics, are explored in the Collège de France lecture series.

Foucault is principally a philosopher of power, and he tracks its movements, patterns, and nuanced effects. His investigations are historical and he marks shifts, developments, and sudden reversals in the techniques of power over time. This genealogical approach, developed with reference to the work of Friedrich Nietzsche, is his signature method; I return to it directly in Chapter 3. Historical shifts give rise to new regimes of governance that act variously to produce subjects, institutions, and knowledge. Foucault pays special attention to discourses (the written and the said) when considering the productive relationship between power and knowledge. He also makes the careful move, in studying the eighteenth century and forward, to resist privileging power's negative impacts and to consider, as a matter of priority, power's productive effects (in constructing identities, for example). This is in part a result of his tracing the shift from the regime of sovereign power to the regime of biopolitics and in part his desire to engage a more profound and nuanced reading of power.

The shift from sovereign power to biopolitics (or biopower) is no sudden change; rather, it develops piecemeal over several centuries.[6] Prior to the seventeenth century, Foucault characterizes power through the figure of the sovereign. The sovereign exercises primarily coercive or negative power—what Foucault refers to as the "right of the sword" (2003b, 240). Individual deaths of those in the king's thrall demonstrates his sovereignty; in other words, the sovereign exercises power in and through the power to kill. In *Discipline and Punish*, Foucault describes the grisly fate of the attempted regicide Damiens, tortured and executed publicly in the sixteenth century for his attempt on Louis XV. Damiens' spectacle of death evoked the king's power as spectacle; Damiens' death made the king's power visible (1979).

Yet, the strategy of sovereign power could not meet the challenges of "demographic explosion and industrialization" (Foucault 2003b, 249). With these changes, "far too many things were escaping the old mechanism of the power of sovereignty, both at the top and at the bottom, both at the level of detail and at the mass level" (*ibid.*). While the sovereign was visible in his kingly power, the people remained invisible to power. Further, the exercise of sovereign power requires direct coercive efforts. Two novel movements of power—*disciplinary* and *regulatory*—established the shifts that would eventually develop into a new regime: biopower (2003b, 243 and 249; Lemke 2011, 36).

Disciplinary power focuses on individual bodies and governs individual behavior at a minute level. According to Foucault, this was the first of the two novel movements to appear because it was "easier and more convenient" to engage detail rather than mass behavior (2003b, 250). It appeared in the seventeenth century as surveillance and training. For example, Foucault describes the soldier of the *Ancien Régime*, noting the dictation of the body's articulations: ". . . they will be taught never to fix their eyes on the ground, but to look straight at those they pass . . . to remain motionless until the order is given, without moving the head, the hands, or the feet . . . lastly to march with a bold step, with knee and ham taut, on the points of the feet, which should face outwards" (an ordinance from 1764, as quoted in Foucault 1979, 180) For Foucault, what distinguishes the disciplinary technique is: its scale of control—it deals with bodies individually—the body as the object of control, and the mode of uninterrupted coercion (Foucault 1979, 181). This attention to detail, repeated in multiple social locations, includes timetables, movement, diet, and behavior in daily life. Disciplinary power produces docile bodies (182). Emerging institutions in the eighteenth and nineteenth centuries, such as the prison, the school, and the hospital follow this pattern. The "fundamental reference" of this kind of power is the "meticulously subordinated cogs of a machine" (186).

As an image of disciplinary power, Foucault famously analyzes Bentham's Panopticon, a prison design that upends the asymmetry of visibility in the regime of sovereign power. He calls this a "marvelous machine" and a "cruel, ingenious cage" which "produces homogenous effects of power" (Foucault 1979, 202 and 205). In the Panopticon, which arranges individual cells in a circle around a guard tower placed in the middle, the governed are completely visible while the seat of power is inaccessible. The prisoners do not know when the guard tower is occupied and so do not know when they are observed. As a result, they self-regulate: "He who is subjected to a field of visibility, and who knows it, assumes responsibility for the constraints of power; he makes them play spontaneously upon himself . . . he becomes the principle of his own subjection" (203). Power's panoptic design produces this self-regulation as a positive effect, and power's reach explodes. Visibility is still asymmetrical, but now the all-seeing eye of power is invisible to those upon whom power operates. Indeed, power's operation is also invisible; no physical torture is necessary here, no public beatings—instead, the governed are internally motivated to precisely follow mandated behavior in order to access a system of rewards and avoid punishment.

Starting in the nineteenth century, another technique of power emerges: *regulatory* power, which deals with life itself and general processes (Foucault 2003b, 249–250). This pattern of power eschews the individual in favor of the population, focusing on birth rate, death rate, disease, and other collective principles. In sum, it "brings together the mass effects characteristic of a population" and seeks to control and predict "the series of random events that can occur in a living mass" (249). Because of its point of application at the level of the mass, it involves significant "coordination and centralization" and the development of knowledge in emerging fields like statistics and epidemiology (Foucault 2003b, 250, cf. Lemke 2011, 5). Regulatory power is interested in homeostasis, balance, and predictability as a mode of governance, which "protects the security of the whole from internal dangers" (Foucault 2003b, 249). For regulatory power (and for biopower in turn) enemies and threats are internal rather than external. Chance and death haunt this power from the inside while power seeks to secure the population and eliminate risk (244). In the same way, enhancement literature construes the human population as internally threatened by vulnerability and interdependence.

The two technologies—disciplinary and regulatory—are not in competition, but rather mutually constitute each other (Lemke 2011, 37). Foucault uses the example of a town, with its various interventions toward governance through health insurance, pensions, hygiene, procreation, and child care, and all the mechanisms and codifications around these interventions, to show that the two technologies are intertwined (2003b, 251). Regulatory and disciplinary techniques are both focused on the body, but one treats the body as an individual and the other "replaces" the body with "general biological processes" (249). Sex is an example of an "apparatus" through which the two technologies of power are jointly expressed (Lemke 2011, 38).

Regulatory power again expands the reach and interests of power. In combination with disciplinary power, regulatory power brings biopower to fruition. Importantly for this book, the two technologies, regulatory and disciplinary, are linked through the *norm* and produce a normalizing society governed by biopower with the body at the center (Foucault 2003b, 253). Rather than the "binary legal code" of the sovereign and the notion of *right*, biopower relies on the norm and engages the "relative logic of calculating, measuring, and comparing" (Lemke 2011, 38–39). This system and its points of application in issues such as sex and health produces, for example, the hereditary theory of degeneracy. Further, it situates medicine as a "power-knowledge" which can work on both the level of the individual and the level of the population with the norm as a hinge between the two (Foucault 2003b, 252).[7] According to Foucault, biopower has "taken control of life in general—with the body as one pole and the population as the other" (253). Recall my construal of bioethics as an organ of biopower, a social location in which the logic of the norm and power-knowledge bear down on individuals and populations like persons with disabilities and women.

While sovereign power is the right of the sword, that is, the power to kill, biopower is the power to make live (Foucault 2003b, 241; cf. Lemke 2011, 36). Yet, the two are layered together rather than neatly divided in history. This means that sovereign power, the taking of life, must still find expression within the regime of biopower. For Foucault, this "death drive" within biopower is *racism* (Foucault 2003b, 254). This produces a "break between what must live and what must die" and is "a way of fragmenting the field of the biological that power controls" (254–255).[8] The racism at the heart of biopolitics, the ability to mark out individuals for death in a system of power built to produce and maintain life (or refuse to maintain it), is precisely where I seek to locate an analysis of disability's role in enhancement literature. The racism at the heart of biopower focuses on the body; it treats the body it discovers as abnormal through the logic of calculation and comparison, and then situates that body as risk for the population. In just the same way, enhancement literature frames disability as risk, undercutting sophisticated and nuanced understandings of disability as social and political in favor of biological reductions.

For Foucault, the biopolitical logic of racism is grounded in the idea that "if you want to live, the other must die" (2003b, 255). More specifically, the logic runs as follows: "the more inferior species die out, the more abnormal individuals are eliminated, the fewer degenerates there will be in the species as a whole, and the more I—as species rather than individual—can live, the stronger I will be, the more vigorous I will be. I will be able to proliferate" (255). As I discuss and analyze the conceptual heart of enhancement literature, we will find that transhumanist thought and strong enhancement enthusiasm seeks security from risk, especially internal risk, and supports the idea that the elimination of some will support the strength of the whole ("as species rather than individual"). While transhumanism seeks maximization, the suggested methods and suggestions related to this maximization reveal an overriding concern with risk and marking out fit and unfit traits. This implies that homeostasis, rather than maximization, may be the practical effect of suggested enhancement techniques. In my analysis of transhumanism in Chapter 1 and in a case study of genetic selection in Chapter 4 I discuss these matters in detail.

I have so far suggested that bioethics and literature on enhancement, like the power-knowledge of medicine more generally, is a product and organ of biopolitics, and that disability is central to this discourse. I have described biopolitics as a regime of power. This contemporary pattern of power functions through the norm, dividing populations between normal and abnormal in order to govern and engage in security measures against risk to manage risk. In this book, I will challenge the identification of disability with risk and describe the ways in which the theoretical commitments I challenge put persons with disabilities at risk. Insofar as enhancement literature attempts to ask and answer the question of who should live, biopolitics is at significant play, and persons with disabilities are marked out for elimination.

In general, my study of enhancement enthusiasm engages a thoroughgoing Foucauldian perspective which takes into account the portrait of power as biopower and borrows liberally from feminist and disability studies. In the pages that follow, I draw attention away from abstract calls for a brighter future and point to the spaces, discourses, and practices of enhancement that exclude and attempt to eliminate disability and demean those with disabilities. I uncover the material reality of the transhumanist utopian vision. The utopia makes itself known through inversion: transhumanists seek to manage risk so the posthuman can be invulnerable; transhumanists seek to control embodiment so the posthuman intellect can roam free.

The five chapters of this book treat the three conceptual threads already evident in this Introduction: enhancement, risk, and disability. In Chapter 1, "Dragon Slayers: Exploring Transhumanism," I cut through philosophical literature on enhancement and belie the common idea that today there are two ideologically opposed camps on the subject—so-called bio-conservatives and bio-liberals. Contemporary philosophers discussing enhancement share multiple key assumptions, a fact that calls into question polarization among academics with regard to the acceptability of enhancement. I uncover the shape and tone of the general conversation regarding enhancement, situate transhumanism within it, and move to engage transhumanist Nick Bostrom at length. Bostrom, in a move representative of the debates, implicitly endorses the idea that political and social problems can be solved through bodily interventions. He specifies that posthumanity—that is, a new and better way to live—is possible if choice is maximized and life thereby unfolds in an open field, unencumbered by the needs of the body. Disability is a matter of chance that must be brought to heel. Being open to chance is characterized as risky and imagined to hold us back from new achievements. This means that the disabled subject is distorted in this discourse as the bearer of risk, presenting it like a virus to the general population, which is called to engage in quarantine. I also engage Julian Savulescu on risk and disability.

To lay the groundwork for continued engagement with enhancement literature, I work against the reduction of disability to a biological matter in Chapter 2, "Rethinking Disability: Dodging Definitions, Muddying Models," and advocate for a Foucauldian-inspired *cultural* reading of the many meanings of disability. Foucault explores the construction of the subject by way of its exclusions in *Discipline and Punish* (1979) and *Abnormal* (2003a). With this understanding of the social construction of the subject in mind, I claim that disability is significantly socially constructed, but exceeds the bounds of identity as a floating sign of deviance. This excess outstrips the "social model" and pushes the broader, cultural reading I advocate. While the disability community is often strategically viewed as a minority group, which like other marginalized groups seeking civil rights and equal treatment, it is important to avoid the pitfalls of that model. A "minority model" may lock persons with disabilities into competition with other marginalized groups and conscript them into participation in policing the border between disability and ability. I assess these models and others to explore the consequences of different ways of thinking "disability." A cultural reading of disability can handle the plasticity and multiplicity of disability's meanings and moments. I will conclude that the view of disability as merely biological, common among transhumanists and within bioethics literature as a whole, is misguided. This view belies political and social solutions to issues raised by disability and encourages turning toward biomedical interventions instead. Enhancement thinking engages disability through the biopolitical frame of biological risk.

In Chapter 3, "Rethinking Enhancement: A Genealogical Approach," I engage in the cultural reading of disability I advocate and explicate in Chapter 2 and push for a biopolitical reading of enhancement enthusiasm. In this chapter, I examine enhancement strategies popular at different moments of the twentieth century. This reading combines the Foucauldian strategies of building genealogy and tracking the play between norm and deviance in biopolitical terms. A Foucauldian genealogy is a material history of the body in which the jolts and chance of history are revealed, rather than an idealized origin point. My genealogy of enhancement enthusiasm tells a story about the relationship between meanings of disability and meanings of enhancement, which move in tandem as a pair and build notions of abnormality along the way. I examine physical culture at the turn of the twentieth century, the birth of the field of endocrinology in the 1910s and 1920s, and, finally, post–Second World War rehabilitations of eugenic thinking in the 1950s. In each of these cultural moments, deviant bodies are assessed and rejected based on then-current modes of conceptualizing health. In light of this history, I argue that contemporary transhumanism, touted as transformative thinking, is not a radical discourse at all but merely repeats the mistakes of the past. Transhumanism replaces previous biological reductions with a specifically *genetic* reduction, but the biopolitical pattern of the discourse of the previous century is maintained. I end the chapter by outlining genetic determinism to better understand the problems in transhumanist thought. While some transhumanists have explicitly rejected genetic determinism as faulty, they implicitly support it rhetorically and practically.

In Chapter 4, "Choosing, for Choice's Sake: A Case Study," I complete my shift back to present-day meanings of both enhancement and disability in a critical analysis of Julian Savulescu's call to employ genetic selection as a moral duty to future generations. His moral principle of "procreative beneficence" urges those considering reproduction to apply evolving technologies as they emerge to create the "best" child possible with the greatest future options (2001b). The desire to maximize choice, to prise open the future for children, plays out as an injunction against using embryos "marked" by positive tests for particular traits—those associated with disability, risk, chance. Again, biopolitical thinking requires pitting the success of the whole population against risks presented by particular "abnormal" individuals. I challenge Savulescu's principle and cry foul with regard to the unqualified good of maximizing choice and the feasibility of reducing chance. I also characterize the move to genetic selection as an expression of genetic bias, an instance of creeping genetic determinism in transhumanist literature, and expose the reduction of disability to genetic profiles.

Fixed: The Science/Fiction of Human Enhancement, a 2013 documentary by independent filmmaker Regan Brashear, depicts some who believe in a burgeoning alliance between transhumanists and disabled persons. Some promote radical enhancement as a path toward fighting disability oppression. With my analysis of Savulescu's enhancement strategy in mind, I end the chapter by calling into question moves transhumanists make in claiming themselves as allies in the fight for disability rights and persons with disabilities as their compatriots in the use of evolving technologies. Given the present form of enhancement enthusiasm, and its lineage traced through enhancement discourse in the last century, any claims to an alliance between transhumanism and disability are, at best, misleading.

I complete my account of the insidious double link between disability and risk in Chapter 5, "Disability as/at Risk: The Biopolitics of Disability." I show that prenatal testing and screening practices, along with genetic counseling, require parents and potential parents to engage in risk management as an attempt to control the future. A look to these practices reveals the disciplinary movement of the call to risk assessment and risk mitigation produces subjectivity as risk management. This subjectivity resonates with the transhumanist characterizations of disability as risk and embodiment as fundamentally vulnerable. It also ensures the hinge between disciplinary and regulatory power, the circulation of the norm, and therefore the governance of biopower. The linkage of disability and risk among enhancement enthusiasts, in discourses surrounding reproductive technology, and in popular media puts those with disabilities at mortal risk. We become used to the linkages and turn away when persons with disabilities, like 14-year-old Alex Spourdalakis, are killed by their families ("ASAN calls" 2013). In other words, the very desire transhumanists express to eliminate risk produces and assigns risk to particular persons, a conceptual scheme that buttresses cultural devaluation of persons with disabilities. When disabled lives are devalued and called into question, and health care and social supports are eliminated or unavailable, persons with disabilities are directly harmed. I conclude that claims regarding the special relationship between risk and disability are spurious. The practice of risk management, whether theoretical or actual, redoubles risk; envisioning a utopia without risk supports risky spaces that literally kill and victimize particular persons.

The enhancement strategies supported by transhumanist visions rely on lethal misinterpretations of enhancement, risk, and disability. Enhancement enthusiasts dream of an extended and autonomous subject who is invulnerable, independent, and can choose from life plans across a maximized range of opportunity. In the transhumanist perspective, all existing persons are found wanting in these respects. But, this evaluation runs contrary to the ethical insights of feminism and disability theory; I would subvert the twinned logics of mastery and autonomy in favor of viewing human life as fundamentally vulnerable and interdependent in valuable ways. The transhumanist desire to radicalize human *shape* through various enhancement strategies leaves untouched the Enlightenment vision of the human being as a floating intellect, trapped and threatened by the body. Indeed, transhumanist thinkers point to Enlightenment thinkers as theoretical ancestors; transhumanism makes radical promises but engages in regressive thinking.

NOTES

1. Foucault refers variously and apparently synonymously to biopower and biopolitics, and it is difficult to tease out a reliable distinction between the two terms (see Lemke 2011, 34, for a full discussion). In this work, I will treat biopower and biopolitics as synonymous.

2. The authors do not believe moral enhancement is likely to supplant moral education entirely, but rather augment it (2012, 11, and 121). But they position it as a necessary addition. They also suggest a political strategy, greatly increased surveillance, in order to meet the problem of terrorism (5). But, according to Persson and Savulescu, liberal societies will resist this strategy and so the need arises again for moral enhancement among voters (98). I return to their argument in Chapter 1.

3. There is some debate over whether these figures count as transhumanists, or merely fellow travelers. Given the content of their work, the fact that Bostrom has readily used the label of transhumanism, and the use of that label in Savulescu's published work, I believe it is fair to refer to them as such and that this label lends clarity when analyzing their positions. I explore this matter further in Chapter 1.

4. In working with the link between risk and identity, I echo Jasbir Puar, who seeks to situate identity as "risk coding" (2009).

5. I use the phrase "already-existing persons" to refer, minimally, to children and adults with disabilities, or persons with dependencies similar to or resonant with what we tend to refer to as disability, whose survival and well-being is called into question by this discourse. Maximally, the phrase can be understood to refer to any child or adult. Later, I use this phrase in connection with a discussion of reproductive liberty and genetic selection. Importantly, this phrase should *not* be understood to refer to an embryo or fetus. For more discussion, see Chapters 2 and 4.

6. This shift does not mean that biopolitics replaces sovereignty as a mode of power, but rather that biopolitics layers over sovereignty, augmenting it and working in tandem with it. Thomas Lemke describes the two as existing simultaneously and that sovereign power is freed from its boundaries by biopower (Lemke 2011, 39).

7. Power-knowledge marks the mutual constitution of power and knowledge. Foucault uniquely engages knowledge as a product of power, rather than the other way around.

8. For a full discussion of racism and biopower, see Bernasconi 2010.

Chapter 1

Dragon Slayers

Exploring Transhumanism

A dragon lives outside the city. No matter what joy, successes, or relationships develop in the city, all who live here know that directly outside of its borders lies a furious monster. This monster salivates, hungry for us. Our city is full of people who love each other and want the best for each other, but something has gone wrong here. For some reason—perhaps fear, perhaps misdirected concerns and the resulting waste of energy—we have all agreed to pay the dragon tribute rather than attempt to kill it. The tribute comes in the form of our loved ones, sent every day to the dragon's maw. The sacrifices we send spare no family and cause enormous grief in this happy place. Why would we refuse to slay the dragon? Some of us, brave and fighting complacency, want to attempt it. The danger of making that attempt is not greater than the tribute that we regularly pay in human flesh. Yet, established powers undercut any plans for dragon slaying. The dragon is an old threat, and we have become used to it. Yes, it hurts badly when we send tribute and lose our loved ones, and we all know our own day is coming to be fed to the monster, but being sent in the dragon's maw is an everyday part of life.

This is the "The Fable of the Dragon-Tyrant"—a parable written by Nick Bostrom, Professor of Philosophy and Director of the Future of Humanity Institute at Oxford University (2005a). Bostrom is a provocative philosopher and the co-founder of the World Transhumanist Association, a network for academics and non-academics alike.[1] For Bostrom, transhumanism stands for the "radical extension of human health-span, eradication of disease, elimination of unnecessary suffering, and augmentation of human intellectual, physical, and emotional capacities . . ." (2005b, 5). The hero of Bostrom's story is the one who finally hatches a plan to slay the dragon, which represents death, and succeeds. Bostrom advocates in the parable for the moral necessity of developing anti-aging technology in the hopes of preventing or postponing death. For Bostrom, death is not something fundamental to life or embodiment, but rather a threat which is utterly excessive and unjust. Death is a dragon-tyrant. To call death a dragon is to claim that it is foreign and hideous, another being that acts upon our bodies. To call death a tyrant is to claim that it is a threat to freedom—that freedom does not thrive where death holds power, and that no one can be free until death is destroyed. For Bostrom, we are wrong and indeed morally complacent to think of death as a fixed part of life.

More generally, Bostrom would like us to recalibrate our sense of what counts as a threat. Although we mourn our friends and loved ones when they die, and often rage against their deaths, whether or not we see a death as wrong or even meaningless depends on contingent factors. For instance, deaths that result from police brutality, or deaths from neglect and abuse, count as injustices. In other words, we have a sense that something has gone wrong, which prepares us to zero in on threats that need to be vanquished. But, we do not typically react this way to all deaths, and Bostrom thinks this is a problem. In a TED talk given in 2005, he compared the loss of a life to the loss of knowledge—a loss at an estimated rate of one book per person. The cost of lost lives due to death, then, he casts as a tragedy akin to the burning of the library at Alexandria, but at a rate of three times per year (2005d).

In this chapter, I consider Bostrom's perspective along with those of other enhancement enthusiasts who, like him, believe that we must take up human enhancement as a global project at the risk of great injustice. From these perspectives, it appears that death is not a fixed part of life—life and death are detachable, and death is a foreign threat to life. Further, it seems, we can measure the value of human life by way of knowledge—individual human beings are valuable because they contribute knowledge to a global library. Yet, death seems immanent to life—cell death occurs regularly in our bodies, and indeed we die even as we live. We live with and in the awareness of our death, even if we reject it stringently. Further, the view that knowledge production is the reason human lives are valuable, or even the primary reason human lives are valuable, is at best a partial and misleading picture and, at worst, dangerous and deadly for those excluded. If one concedes that knowledge is what makes life valuable, this implies that persons whose knowledge is discounted or disqualified—people with intellectual disabilities, along with other vulnerable people around the globe—do not have lives worth living. Contesting this caricature of human life is part of the project of this book.

In this chapter, I ground my critique of transhumanism by exploring the debate over enhancement in today's bioethics literature and situating transhumanist views within that literature. I go on to engage Nick Bostrom and Julian Savulescu, whose work I characterize as transhumanist. Clarifying what human enhancement is will be tricky, as the definition of enhancement is often contested.

CONTEMPORARY DEBATE

To hazard a starting point, enhancement refers to the pursuit or use of medical and technological strategies to augment human traits. Augmentation can be achieved through a variety of means, from shoes and caffeine to neural implants and prosthetics. This makes enhancement a loose concept. Indeed, for some proponents of enhancement, the moral acceptability of novel enhancement strategies stems directly from their supposed similarity to everyday activities of improvement, such as learning. Bioethicist John Harris claims that enhancement is good and desirable by definition; according to him, "if it wasn't good for you it wouldn't be enhancement" (2011, 131). But, we should refuse to beg the moral question, as Harris does here. One cannot assume that enhancement is morally acceptable without, in effect, refusing to enter the debate before it begins.

So, how can enhancement be morally evaluated? Problems crop up immediately. Ethically separating strength training and steroids, for example, seems to require uneasy notions of the natural or the authentic, wherein strength training is morally acceptable while steroids involve cheating. But, the line does not hold. Strength training and the ingestion of steroids both induce the body to react to newly introduced environmental conditions that would not otherwise occur. In the larger scheme of things, how does one react, for example, when a person's sense of the authentic is not born out through one's embodied experience, as in the case of those who identify as transgender? Meanwhile, the invocation of the long-contested divide between therapy and enhancement could separate reconstructive plastic surgery from cosmetic plastic surgery. The line does not hold here, either, as it depends on the treatment of the species-typical body as normative and this in turn depends on the historically contingent and fluctuating diagnoses of medical professionals. Some philosophers use these two distinctions, between the authentic and the unauthentic and between therapy and enhancement, to maintain that only authentic or therapeutic enhancements are morally acceptable, thereby taking much of what proponents of enhancement mean when they use the word "enhancement" off the table. Others, like Harris, forego these distinctions to argue that all enhancements—globally—are not only morally acceptable but also morally obligatory.

Harris does, however, reference the difference between negative eugenics, which aims to cure diseases and prevent so-called birth defects, and positive eugenics, which aims, in Harris's words, to make "better people" (2007). But, Harris himself covers over this distinction when he writes:

> The moral motive for using technology to intervene in the natural lottery of life is for the sake of the goods that this will bring about . . . equality of opportunity may sometimes be one of these goods . . . saving lives or what is the same thing, postponing death, removing or preventing disability or disease or enhancing human functioning are the more obvious and usually the more pressing reasons. (2011, 147)

This passage conflates "removing or preventing disability or disease" and "enhancing human functioning." In practice, the distinction between positive and negative eugenics is just as misleading as other common divides. The commonplace view that disability is to be avoided, and to enhance means much the same thing as avoiding disability, means that a disability analysis of enhancement issues is necessary.

Given this, a fruitful way to analyze enhancement in contemporary debate is to redirect our attention to what proponents of enhancement strategies desire and note the position of disability within the discourse. Once the blurred lines between therapeutic interventions or enhancements, negative or positive eugenics are set aside, discussions of the ethics of enhancement are transformed. Debates over enhancement are less about available technology than potential technology deemed worthy of investment on the basis of specific goals. Enhancement proponents are utopian thinkers and their utopias are reflected in concrete recommendations with regard to how we must engage technology to improve our lives and those of our children. Seeing this clearly allows one to situate innovative technologies and weigh what is aimed for by their use. What does the future look like, to the hopeful enhancement enthusiast?

If we focus on enhancement's goals, rather than slippery distinctions, we can critically assess enhancement and avoid begging the moral question of enhancement (i.e. assuming that enhancement is good, full stop). The burden in the debate is thus shifted back to proponents of enhancement, who—as we shall discover—weave fantasies of health, ability, and the good life that are troublesome and exclusionary. Taking this tack, I closely examine the goals of enhancement's primary enthusiasts, the transhumanists I introduced by way of Bostrom's parable. Because I respond to the argumentation of these enthusiasts, I can sharpen my loose definition of enhancement to take up enhancement the way they do: namely, as the practice of adding to, protecting, or maximizing capabilities by way of technological intervention upon the body. I therefore engage what some scholars call *radical enhancement*, which Nicholas Agar (2010) describes as the possibility that medicine, science, and technology would so radically improve various aspects of life that the beings who would result would not be recognizably human.

As discussed in the Introduction, some might complain that transhumanist views are too extreme to offer a fair portrait of enhancement's possibilities and that, therefore, my project in this book is also bound to miss the mark. I have already defended my decision to take on a flawed but influential discourse. But, further, it is worth noting that some more moderate philosophers play it too safe with regard to enhancement. They make proposals with which no one would disagree, such as being sure any proposed enhancement is accessible and effective and that harm to individuals is to be avoided at all costs. These qualifications do not get us any clearer on the special issues presented by the ethical question of enhancement—indeed, they sound like prescriptions for action for any public policy development, and they are subject to the same roadblocks. Finally, buried at the heart of the moderates' safe argumentation is a problem. Among those who engage in the question of enhancement a set of crucial assumptions are shared quite broadly. Ultimately, there is a consensus in bioethics, continuous with transhumanist thought, which should be challenged.

Despite this larger consensus, there is little holding together the haphazard mix of enhancement procedures discussed in bioethics literature. This is not surprising, given the looseness with which enhancement is defined and the troubled distinctions that remain at play. Procedures include technological and medical interventions, both sought-after and already accomplishable. Bioethicists discuss everything from the body-contouring effects of liposuction to scientific research aimed at discovering ways to counteract the aging process in cells. But, emerging technologies, including genetic screening and editing procedures such as CRISPR, capture center stage.[2] Nootropic drugs (cognitive enhancers like modafinil), also receive high levels of attention (Battleday and Brem 2015). So, what is uniquely at stake in contemporary discussions is the acceptability of heritable medical interventions, with special attention to the mind.

The idea of permanent or heritable changes has led bioethicists to either speculate about the exciting novelty available through technology or worry that humanity, or what is important about us, will be irrevocably lost. These responses fall into two groups placed on either end of an ersatz political spectrum: bio-conservatives (called "bioluddites" by transhumanist James Hughes and anti-meliorists by bioethicist Arthur Kaplan) and, opposing them, those who are pro-enhancement. This group is typically referred to as "bio-libertarian" and overlaps significantly with thinkers who consider themselves transhumanists, or at least fellow travelers. Bio-conservatives and bio-libertarians are treated, by those both inside and outside of the debate, as if they were in deep disagreement.

Bio-conservatives blossom from the theological roots of bioethics. Paul Ramsey, one of the first to consider the broader impact of emerging medical technologies, was a theologian and could be cast as the original bio-conservative. He felt comfortable with a distinction between manufacture and procreation, which valorizes the natural or the authentic (1970, 136–137). In response to the work of Francis Crick, Ramsey worried that we sought to produce a man-God hybrid by genetic means who would destroy "the sanctity of the individual" (146). In a twist, the theologian acted as a humanist—he worried about the loss of what makes humanity special. He foresaw species-suicide in a mechanized future (152–153).

Ramsey's worries are picked up by today's bio-conservatives. Leon Kass, who names Ramsey as a mentor, believes we should cede procreative and evolutionary matters to God, gods, or a causal force in a god-like role (1997 and 2002). The Icarus myth is often invoked by those who agree with him. Similarly, thinkers like Jürgen Habermas and Michael Sandel enjoin us to protect the boundaries of human nature, along with human dignity, from interference and temptation. Tied to this are Sandel's appeals, which echo Kass's work, to human wisdom and appropriate humility. Resonating among bio-conservatives is a commonplace claim originally made by Ramsey: "Men ought not to play God before they learn to be men, and after they have learned to be men they will not play God" (1970, 137).

The "playing God" objection is curious because it assumes that technology can give us such total control that we might as well call ourselves God. This is chimerical. But, more curious still is the fact that transhumanists also embrace a portrait of technology that implies God-like control, a move which mystifies and elevates technology (Bostrom 2003). Outsized belief in the power of technology over human life, as if it were a foreign invader, is shared by proponents and opponents of enhancement technologies alike—although, of course, the former think we must embrace it and the latter, reject it. In fact, although arguments which react to and reject, or pursue and embrace, the question of whether enhancement is permissible appear to cut a wide swath of argumentation strategies, "conservative" and "libertarian" responses are actually in lock-step with regard to several assumptions. Beyond the mystification and elevation of technology to a God-like role, otherwise-opposed bioethicists agree on the importance of authenticity, the uniqueness of human beings, and the importance of equal opportunity. This overlap is significant.[3]

First, authenticity; among enhancement's detractors, including Norman Daniels, Carl Elliott, and Sandel, it is assumed that humans rightly seek ways to express their authentic selves—yet, this search can be subverted by enhancement procedures. Erik Parens tracks the prevalence of the issue of authenticity among detractors and supporters alike, noting that both groups attempt to solve problems of self-alienation (2009). Thinking back to Bostrom's parable, consider that he poses death as an obstacle to loving human relationships. Death is an interruption which dissolves communities—so enhancement strategies which subvert death can enhance human communities and our authentic selves in turn. Bostrom argues that the quest for authenticity and respect for human beings should mean following the very human drive toward innovation by embracing change through directed evolution. This includes refusing to accept things like aging and death, which cause great distress to humans (Bostrom 2004 and 2005a). Transhumanists like Bostrom see the refusal to direct evolution as tantamount to anti-humanism.

Second, both sides of the debate claim that the human being is uniquely placed among the things in the natural world. This is an outgrowth of authenticity discussions. For conservative responders, authentic *human* living means respecting the boundaries of what is considered unique to human "nature," which might include or depend upon parenthood, sexual reproduction, or even some nameless X-factor (Fukuyama 2002; Kass 1997 and 2002; Sandel 2007). On this basis, enhancement is rejected as threatening what is valuable about humanity or the social world in which human beings find themselves. Yet Bostrom and transhumanist Anders Sandberg argue that paying attention to human wisdom (as the bio-conservative desires) requires taking enhancement seriously because humans are uniquely situated to draw lessons from history and evolution (Bostrom 2004; Bostrom and Sandberg 2011).

Another touchstone in this debate is equality of opportunity, which is called upon to both justify and object to interventionist medical and technological enhancement strategies. This deepens agreement within the literature by returning to concerns about authenticity and pointing to the importance of fair play and the metaphor of competition. Buchanan *et al.* significantly rely on the importance of equality of opportunity in *From Chance to Choice* (2000). They claim that the arena of justice is, in effect, a phenomenon of slow "colonization" of circumstances once left to chance (82–84). On this view, intervention is only ethically justified when we have control over (have colonized) circumstances, but that realm grows along with new technologies and scientific understanding. This is a technological imperative. That is, as technology becomes available that can be used to intervene upon the human body, one should use it. Buchanan *et al.* justify this imperative via the concept of equal opportunity. The authors use Thomas Scanlon's brute luck conception of justice, which they argue should not be limited to nullifying the inequality resulting from natural or social lotteries. Instead, it should be applied earlier, to the "genetic lottery," in order to remain consistent with its claims regarding justice and equality of opportunity (108–152). Of interest for the continued discussion in this book is the implication that the growth of arenas of control is potentially without limit, and that outside of those arenas only chance operates.

Meanwhile, Peter Singer invokes equal opportunity to discuss possible negative effects of enhancement, specifically genetic interventions. He claims that genetic intervention would work against equal opportunity unless it is regulated (2011). This is because of its potential, in a global marketplace, to be used only by already-advantaged persons with ready access to wealth. Because enhancement via genetic intervention is hoped to be heritable, the advantages the wealthy enjoy over the poor would be solidified through the passing of advantageous traits to descendants, widening the gap between rich and poor (cf. Silver 1998). Echoing Singer on this point, Francis Fukuyama claims that transhumanism is the world's most dangerous idea (2004). Solidified advantages enjoyed by the wealthy over the poor violate equal opportunity.

So far, then, three shared concepts among those in the debate over enhancement are uncovered. These shared assumptions already belie the supposedly diametric opposition between two camps on the question of enhancement. But, a fourth fundamental assumption among enhancement scholars eclipses the others and is most important for my discussion in this book, because it firmly places both camps within the same interpretive stance. This final assumption is that complex social and political circumstances, along with hope for change, can be reduced to one dimension—the *biological*.

In biological reductions, relevant information about individual or social circumstances are read through features and facts about the body. For example, the debate over cloning—supposedly divisive—is dictated on both sides by biological reductionism, as Jacques Derrida points out (2005). On the one hand, some have argued that cloning is an affront to human dignity, because it inhibits a kind of right to be an individual. But, arguments of this kind elevate the importance of replicated DNA material to the level of identity. On the other hand, to argue that cloning is a technological innovation of key importance for future change engages the body as a site of political problem-solving. Further, advocates of the use of cloning technology strictly separate reproduction via cloning from typical reproduction, which also signals a kind of misunderstanding—reproduction, as Derrida contends, is always a matter of repetition, and cloning will always involve novel elements (146–148).

Debates over genetic modification technologies are plagued by a particular kind of biological reduction—that is, a causal reduction: genetic determinism. Again we see remarkable consensus among those in bioethics, which—as I will show—extends significantly to transhumanist thinkers. In a review of the literature, David Resnik and Daniel Vorhaus point out that four central objections to genetic modification are based in or influenced by genetic determinism (2006). These are: the freedom argument, which claims that genetic modification interferes with human freedom; the giftedness argument, which claims that children will become products rather than gifts; the authenticity argument, which claims that "talents and abilities" resulting from modification are not really one's own; and the uniqueness argument, which claims that clones are persons whose uniqueness has been violated. Each of these arguments is based on an overestimation of the value of genetic factors.

Yet, arguments advocating for genetic modification to achieve a variety of goals fall into the same traps. Hughes' essay "The Struggle for a Smarter World" promotes cognitive enhancement (2008). Hughes links intelligence to genetics with reference to twin studies and studies of predictors for intelligence among affluent children (943–944). For him, humans have reached the limits of their intellectual potential sans genetic intervention; even when children have access to privileges and advantages their peers do not have, the studies he cites are meant to show that genetics still play a role. But, the portrait of genetic influence Hughes works with is too strong. Arguments supporting programs of genetic enhancement are automatically susceptible to the charge of genetic determinism. This is because making public policy recommendations that would dedicate a vast sum of funds to create genetic enhancement technologies and make them available to the public at least approaches what Mianna Lotz refers to as "geneticism"—the privileging of genetic causes over other factors—if not a stronger variety of genetic determinism (Lotz 2008).

Genetic determinism has two inflections. The first reads as follows: if a trait is identified as genetically or biologically determined, it is unchangeable (or opportunities to alleviate it are significantly limited), and responsibility for the issue falls to the individual rather than political or social institutions (Haslam 2011, 819; Lewontin 1992, 23, 36–37; Nelkin and Lindee 1995, 16, 18, 93). Consider the case of allergies or genetic predispositions to certain sensitivities that would rule out a person working in certain environments. Rather than ensuring safe working conditions in a workplace, the employer has recourse to require a person to disclose any sensitivities and then can declare the worker not fit for the workplace (as opposed to the workplace being unfit for workers) (Nelkin and Lindee 1995, 161). The second inflection suggests that if a trait is genetically determined it is changeable, but only through technology or genetic interventions (Nelkin and Lindee 1995, 101). In a genetic reduction, a genetic problem requires a genetic or technological—rather than a social or political—solution. For example, we might "select against" an embryo carrying an unwanted genetic trait. I return to this strategy as my case study in Chapter 4, and use it to point to the practical conflation of positive and negative eugenics.

Although biological reductions appear throughout bioethics literature, they are particularly prominent among transhumanists. Creeping genetic determinism among transhumanists sets the stage to judge quality of life through genetic profiles. Transhumanists who work in the genetic mode render the body, taken as a bundle of genes, the primary site of human (and therefore, social and political) improvement while at the same time taking for granted that technological interventions on the body, especially genetic interventions, have the power to "enhance" (as Singer does, above). This disregards political and social responsibility for quality of life.

In sum, supposedly diametrically opposed positions in bioethical debates over enhancement actually share fundamental presuppositions. By focusing on shared assumptions, I historicize and contextualize the debate over enhancement. This work only accentuates the need to philosophically investigate the goals of enhancement with more care and rigor. Other oddities in the literature are revealed with close readings; for example, the privileging of male and Western perspectives in the debate. Take the pressure to be tall and deliberation regarding the use and distribution of the human growth hormone to the end of tallness (see Daniel Brock and Eric Juengst in Parens 1998; Buchanan *et al.* 2000, 115–119). The example is usually posed as a problem among young boys. Use of this example to discuss possible enhancements obfuscates and trivializes the bodily stigma and pressure to conform felt by those whose bodies have been raced, sexed, and disabled. Relatedly, the motive to enhance is often characterized by many male bioethicists as an issue of competition, which is already obvious from worries over fair play (Buchanan *et al.* 2000, 74). Overall, we need to enhance the conversation regarding enhancement in order to engage in moral assessment.

TRANSHUMANISM AND ITS GOALS

While the commitments I explore are widely shared across the spectrum of critical debate over enhancement, transhumanists are particularly frank about their assumptions as they work to promote enhancement. Their transparency provides an entry point for the critical engagement in this book. But, because transhumanism assumptions are widespread, my critique can be applied to larger currents in bioethics. I now turn to read transhumanism more closely and begin to tell the story of the desire for enhancement. What future do transhumanists hope to bring about through enhancement technologies? I look to transhumanist goals in order to understand enhancement enthusiasm.

Transhumanists extol the potential achievements of evolving technology, the desirability of developing new technology, and the possibility of enhancing current human capabilities (Bostrom 2005b, 8). Transhumanism is a multidisciplinary applied ethics. According to the "Transhumanist Declaration," penned in 1998 as a founding document of the World Transhumanist Association, transhumanists recognize that technology has the power to impact human life in a fundamental way that would "redesign" it (Bostrom 2005b, Appendix). Instead of turning away from technology or indulging in "technophobia," (the mistake of bio-luddites) transhumanists believe that new technologies in the fields of genetics, robotics, information, and nanotechnology—should be welcomed as potentially improving human life, although they are risky (*ibid.*, see also Garreau 2005, 115; Rubin 2008, 137). Transhumanist promote the investment of time and research into technology to improve cognition, anti-aging techniques, reproductive technology, and life suspension techniques such as cryogenics—all of which are cited by the Declaration—in order to understand both their risks and possibilities. Ultimately, what individuals stand to gain, according to transhumanists, is the "use of technology to extend their mental and physical (including reproductive) capacities and to improve their control over their own lives" (Bostrom 2005b, Appendix). In sum, the Declaration claims that transhumanists "seek personal growth beyond our current biological limitations" (*ibid.*).

In a 2005 essay, Bostrom traces a history of transhumanism. Taking literary epics, ceremony, and religion as a guide, he notes that cultures around the world have long bemoaned death and sought immortality. He regards Renaissance humanism and the Enlightenment as primary precursors of today's transhumanist point of view, because, like transhumanism, both of these historical frames emphasized the intellect and relied upon empiricism and human judgment to investigate the world and its possibilities, therefore eschewing dogma (2005b, 2). Following Francis Bacon, Bostrom argues that science should be used to "achieve mastery over nature in order to improve the living conditions of human beings" (*ibid.*, see also Rubin 2008, 137). In short, "rational humanism" is where transhumanism locates its heritage, adding only that the human is among those objects of nature to be conquered (Bostrom 2005b, 3).

It is a reading of Immanuel Kant's motto "Sapere aude! Have courage to use your own intelligence!" to which Bostrom finally turns (2005b, 4; cf. Wolfe 2009, xiv). In accordance with Bostrom's vision, the reshaping of the human being would be directed toward improvement in terms of *capabilities*, but also, in harmony with John Stuart Mill, *happiness* (2005b, 4). Transhumanism's hoped-for, reshaped human being is often referred to as the *posthuman*. According to the "Transhumanist FAQ," a collectively authored document Bostrom participated in: "Posthumans could be completely synthetic artificial intelligences, or they could be enhanced uploads . . . or they could be the result of making many smaller but cumulatively profound augmentations to a biological human" (*Humanity* + 2012). To be posthuman, according to transhumanists, is to inhabit a state generally considered not only a departure from what are commonly considered human qualities but also radically better than, or transcendent of, humanity as we know it (Bostrom 2008).

Human-machine hybridity is already a reality in the use of prosthetics, computers, handheld devices, assistive technologies, and other complex technological systems upon which most of us rely every day (cf. Francis 2009 on complex cognition). For more obvious radical examples of hybridity, look to world-class athlete Aimee Mullins, whose 12 pairs of prosthetic legs gained fame in a popular TED talk (2009). One may thus argue, along with Donna Haraway, that we are already posthuman. But, here I am concerned with investigating the transhumanist promotion of a specific, hoped-for, future posthuman, believed by transhumanists to be so increased in capacities that it would be difficult to assign the word "human" to this being.

There are a variety of senses of posthumanism. Transhumanism's sense of the *posthuman* is not the only contemporary meaning of the term, and distinguishing among various meanings of posthumanism will help illuminate transhumanism's usage. Transhumanism's posthuman is not equivalent, for instance, to the concept of posthuman used in critical animal studies to challenge philosophical investments in or the moral relevance of traditional species boundaries. For example, in *What is Posthumanism?* Cary Wolfe forcefully distinguishes transhumanism from the critical posthumanism he endorses. Wolfe draws this line precisely because he recognizes the humanism that Bostrom identifies as the "roots" of transhumanism, a sense of "posthumanism [that] derives directly from ideals of human perfectibility, rationality, and agency" (Wolfe 2009, xiii). Wolfe uses his own posthumanist critique to target these ideals, and to show that the positive "aspirations" of humanism are "undercut by the philosophical and ethical frameworks used to conceptualise them" (xvi). Among these aspirations are better treatment of nonhuman animals and persons with disabilities that the confining "normative subjectivity" of humanism prevents (xvi–xvii). Wolfe compares posthumanism to transhumanism in this way: "posthumanism in my sense isn't posthuman at all—in the sense of being 'after' our embodiment has been transcended—but is only posthuman*ist*, in the sense that it opposes the fantasies of disembodiment and autonomy, inherited from humanism itself . . ." (xv). In contrast, Bostrom's vision of the posthuman is a realization of the fantasies of disembodiment and autonomy and so supports, rather than questions, normative subjectivity.

A version of posthumanism has been attributed to Foucault because of his remark that the human being, as known to us, is a recent invention that may soon be left behind or die out (Foucault 1973, 386–87). I linger here because of the importance of Foucault's work for my project. But, Foucault's sense of posthumanism would amount to the recognition that discourse and power relations always shape human identity, which can shift and be refashioned. Unlike Bostrom, who considers the intellect trapped in the body (an inheritance from Plato, who suggested the same thing about the soul), Foucault believed that the soul is the "prison of the body" (Foucault 1979, 30). Arnold Davidson, in an introduction to the *Abnormal* lectures, explains that Foucault provides a "historical analysis" and "political history" of the body by focusing on the ways that the concepts of the psyche and personality came about, contributing to "gradation from normal to abnormal" in the classification of bodies (Davidson, in Foucault 2003a, xix). But, Foucault investigated and uncovered systems of subject-making and normalization precisely because he was a critic of Enlightenment humanism (Sawicki 1994, 288). Foucault theorized that evolving concepts of the human structure acceptance and rejection of particular bodies, and contribute to suspect normalization practices. Meanwhile, transhumanist thinking serves to further buttress notions of abnormality that are in turn used to exclude certain bodies from political and social privileges.

Despite rallying around a vision of the posthuman, transhumanism is not identical with the ironic cyborg utopia first imagined by Donna Haraway in 1985. Haraway is another philosopher of posthumanism and the author of "The Cyborg Manifesto" (1991), an iconic essay of political ironism in which she imagines border crossings that break oppressive dualisms and acknowledges that human beings are already chimeras and cyborgs. Wolfe identifies Haraway's legacy as the "cyborg" strand of posthumanism and claims that although transhumanism takes cues from her work, it does not much resemble the spirit of Haraway's attempted intervention (2009, xiii). Transhumanism looks forward to a time when posthumans arrive, but Haraway's work argues that distinctions which uphold the figure of the human as autonomous, whole, and rational are already broken down and inapplicable.[4]

Bostrom provides a robust defense of his vision of posthumanity (2009). He lays out the case for posthumanism in the transhumanist sense of having "vastly greater capacities than present human beings have," and marks nature as a work-in-progress (619). He denies that transhumanism entails technological optimism; he takes risk seriously and knows that technology can be misused. Bostrom has referred to this kind of optimism as the "Panglossian view," which he uses to refer to the mistaken idea that progress will reliably continue apace as it has in the past (2004). He refuses to engage in "punishable hubris" (2009, 620). But, he also seeks a proactive stance toward technology and refuses the reactive stance of worries over playing God. Bostrom begins with the premise that we have biological limitations which are so familiar to us that they are easy to overlook; yet, medicine and technology can be applied to move or overcome these limits (*ibid.*).

Our limitations are various, but they include the kinds of biological limitations often attributed to animals and even "the capacity to form a realistic intuitive understanding of what it would be like to be a radically enhanced human" (2009, 620).[5] We lack this capacity because the posthuman is an erstwhile human with radically increased capacities. Bostrom argues that the opportunity range of a posthuman is larger in scope than that of a human. These ranges can be represented by two concentric circles, with the posthuman opportunity range encompassing that of the human (2009, 620, cf. 2008). An opportunity range is an idealized set of possibilities based on available capacities; as defined by bioethicist Norman Daniels, an opportunity range is "the array of life plans reasonable persons . . . are likely to construct for themselves" (Daniels 1985, 33). Bostrom claims that increased opportunity ranges and the unknown potential of increased intellectual capacity is desirable, although it is currently unknowable to us (2009, 620 and 622).

Other human limitations are our lifespan (as discussed at the outset of this chapter), which Bostrom believes currently does not allow enough time for projects or character development, and our intellectual capacity (2009, 620–621). With regard to intellectual capacity, Bostrom worries that our current "cognitive makeup" closes the door to "whole strata of understanding and mental activity" (621). We do not have the brain power to understand every book in the Library of Congress, for example, and most worrisomely, there may be a "cap on our ability to discover philosophical and scientific truths" (*ibid.*). Likening the situation to Plato's cave, Bostrom wonders whether the seeming intractability of major problems in philosophy could be due to the fact that we are not intellectually able to grasp answers to them (*ibid.*).

Bostrom outlines many other human limitations, including in the areas of bodily functionality, sensory modalities, special faculties and sensibilities, and mood, energy, and self-control (2009, 621–622). He desires the ability to protect ourselves from disease, shape our bodies freely, and the freedom offered by copying a version of our brain in silicon (621).[6] These improvements in bodily functionality would improve our quality of life (*ibid.*). With regard to the human senses, he seeks "higher levels of sensitivity and responsiveness" (622). With regard to mood and energy, he cites the widely held view that "we often fail to feel as happy as we like" (*ibid.*). The fact that we do not always feel the best possible sensations, or feel as happy as we are in our best moments, is a problem for Bostrom on par with existential risk and death. Unfortunately, most of us are not good at recognizing these issues as problems (2005d). Finally, he claims that we have limited willpower to break habits (2009, 622). He does warn, however, that movements to make bad habits easier to break might impede "the ability to form stable, hard-to-break habits" (*ibid.*). For Bostrom, these types of unintended effects are to be carefully considered and actively avoided.

As aforementioned, Bostrom believes that we can desire the unknowable with regard to the increased capacities of the posthuman. Taking up David Lewis' view of dispositional value, that "something is a value for you if and only if you would want it if you were perfectly acquainted with it," Bostrom suggests that there may be valuable things we do not currently want because we do not know about them and do not have the knowledge necessary to consider them (2009, 622). For him, we can begin to value posthuman existence even from a limited capacity to understand it and on the basis of currently held values (*ibid.*). This implies that we need not choose the posthuman over human life, but some of our ideals are currently not accessible to us. Therefore, transhumanism, in its pursuit of the posthuman, would allow us to "explore hitherto inaccessible realms of value" (623).

While currently available tools are not to be dismissed, Bostrom claims that low-tech means to this exploration, like education, have limits which can be surpassed by technological means. (2009, 623). But, in order to engage technological means to explore the posthuman realm, he sets out several objectives for policy that he sees as "basic conditions" for transhumanist goals (*ibid.*). These include, as a non-negotiable requirement, global security, including the avoidance of existential risk. Existential risk is a situation in which "an adverse outcome would either annihilate Earth-originating intelligent life or permanently and drastically curtail its potential" (*ibid.*). Further, technological progress, augmented by economic growth, is necessary. This is because "aging, disease, feeble memories and intellects, a limited emotional repertoire and inadequate capacity for sustained well-being" are difficult problems to solve (*ibid.*). Finally, he believes it would be "sub-optimal" if wide access to exploration of the posthuman were not possible. He believes there are many good reasons to support wide access to new technologies (623–624).

According to Bostrom, these commitments mean that transhumanists value individual freedom and choice. For him, limitations to bodily modification based on another person's disgust "would not normally be a legitimate ground for coercive interference," and "centrally planned efforts" for making better people are wrong (2009, 624). We should promote democracy the world over in order to aid in responsible decision-making with regard to technology. We cannot rely on "our old habits and beliefs" to make "wise choices" and should further take advantage of the insights of artificial intelligence as it surpasses human intelligence (*ibid.*). Additionally, transhumanists value the well-being of all sentient life, which deserves our consideration as we pursue posthumanism (a concern that becomes all the more urgent, Bostrom implies, if we are successful). Finally, Bostrom emphasizes that we must save lives, as that is of primary moral value; this includes working against involuntary death and aging. For him, as we learned at the outset of this chapter, anti-aging medicine is of primary importance and cryonic suspension should be made available (*ibid.*).

Bostrom recognizes that this picture is not appealing to everyone. He notes that many balk at the idea of these new technologies, especially genetic enhancement technologies, which are central to the conversation, and consider them morally wrong (2012, 108). The outcomes that some worry about, including making children into products and increasing social prejudice against persons with disabilities, would also be bad from a transhumanist perspective (*ibid.*). But, ultimately, Bostrom does not believe that these bad outcomes will come about as a result of the transhumanist pursuit of posthumanity:

> such dystopian scenarios are speculations. There is no firm ground for believing that the alleged consequences would actually happen. What relevant evidence we have, for instance regarding the treatment of children who have been conceived through the use of in vitro fertilization or embryo screening, suggests that the pessimistic prognosis is alarmist. Parents will in fact love and respect their children even when artificial means and conscious choice play a part in procreation. (2012, 108–109)

He further claims that it is possible that parents will find it easier to love children who are happy and healthy, and people with disabilities will be better off. For him, good consequences and bad are both possible, but the "potential gains are enormous . . . healthier, wittier, happier people may be able to reach new levels culturally" (109).

As aforementioned, Bostrom's vision of the pursuit of transhumanist goals does not involve central planning. He believes that one good reason to avoid regulation is past genocidal horror of state-sponsored eugenics programs (2012, 110). He acknowledges, however, that the libertarian approach has drawbacks; specifically, children have important interests that must be considered. But, current measures to protect children can be extended to deal with genetic enhancement technologies and other emerging technologies. He focuses again on risk and opportunities, arguing that "we ought to outlaw genetic modifications that are intended to damage the child or limit its opportunities in life, or that are judged to be too risky" (*ibid.*). Further, if the worry is over access, subsidies can be used for basic enhancements. Mandates, however, should be avoided (*ibid.*). Using subsidies and other forms of encouragement, Bostrom does not want to encourage positional advantage enhancements (like height).[7] Encouraged enhancements should have both significant intrinsic benefits and positive social externalities (like health) (111). Most cases are mixed, like memory and intellect, and in these cases we should weigh the externalities. If the positive externalities are high, we should encourage and subsidize this type of enhancement (depending on the political climate) (112).

Other concerns may arise, such as Fukuyama's widely cited concern that the human species will split into two across already-existing fault lines of inequality (Bostrom 2012, 112; cf. Fukuyama 2002 and 2004). According to Bostrom, some inequalities are unfair, but we don't think all are; therefore, some of the same justifications that allow inequality today could allow inequality that results from germline engineering (112–113). Bostrom is thinking of cases in which inequalities are based on merit, have social benefit, or are the result of foolish decision-making (112). Bad inequality can meanwhile be counteracted with social policies like subsidies or free services; we might also consider mandating net-positive genetic enhancements that would counteract the inequality that arises from free choice (113). But, this may not be necessary; it is very possible that instead of increasing inequality, "the lot of the genetically worst-off is radically improved" (*ibid.*).

Finally, Bostrom acknowledges the issue of the hubris he wants to avoid. He wonders whether, in pursuing posthumanism, we are potentially arrogantly damning future generations to irreversible changes we do not yet understand (2012, 113–114). Germ-line interventions sound much less appealing when human fallibility is in full view (114). Yet, in an argumentative move that rings of simple techno-optimism, Bostrom argues that germ-line interventions can be reversed by other germ-line interventions. These interventions would be more easily undertaken by future, enhanced generations. While we should be careful about the risks of unintended effects on drive and ambition, germ-line interventions are no more objectionable to Bostrom than typical social reforms (*ibid.*).

Overall, Bostrom believes a future of increased happiness is possible if only we were to invest in enhancement technologies—not only a future of new pleasure, but also an increasingly moral and politically just future (Bostrom 2008). Bostrom argues that the posthuman state is better, offering pleasures and fulfillments worth pursuing, although he simultaneously acknowledges that his vision of posthuman life is by definition unknowable to mere humans because it involves the attainment of new capacities and, thus, new insights (2004 and 2008, 112). He writes, as if from the future: "[Posthumans] love life every instant. Every second is so good that it would blow our minds had their amperage not been previously increased" (2010, 8). This point is typical of the rhetorical strategy Bostrom employs. Bostrom contrasts an unknowable future of intense happiness with contemporary conditions, and describes today's world in dismal terms, taking suffering for granted. Both moves seem unjustified. Regarding today, he writes:

> Every way you turn it's the same: soot, casting its veil over all glamours and revelries, despoiling your epiphany, sodding up your white pressed collar and shirt. And once again that familiar beat is audible, the beat of numbing routine rolling along its tracks. The commuter trains loading and unloading their passengers . . . sleepwalkers, shoppers, solicitors, the ambitious and the hopeless,

> the contented and the wretched . . . like human electrons shuffling through the circuitry of civilization. (2010, 2)

Readers are thus exhorted to promote a transhumanist vision of the future. To envision that future, Bostrom asks us to recall the best moments of our lives and hold them in our hearts as an "aspiring ember"; he argues that the best moments of human life correspond with a "higher state of being," the thought of which should provide motivation enough to pursue radical enhancement (2010, 3 and 5).

There is a false dilemma here between control and chance, complacent wretchedness and the heights of happiness. It seems that for transhumanists, only two reactions to technology—that is, passivity and activity—are possible. They trade in one false dilemma, that between techno-optimism and techno-pessimism, for another. Activity is preferable because (or so it is claimed) technology has the potential to ameliorate or eliminate human suffering and put individuals in control, while passivity should be rejected because it may increase, or at least extend, human suffering. Passivity represents ignoring possible control over one's future. From this perspective, it seems that being subject to chance is anti-human (insofar as to be human is to engage proactively with change), anti-happiness, and anti-progressive. Along these lines, many transhumanists dismiss arguments coming from bio-conservatives who they believe opt for passivity. But, characterizing worries about radical enhancement as a refusal to alleviate suffering closes off conversation prematurely; there are, as we shall see, good reasons to worry about enhancement strategies that do not involve the rejection of emerging technologies as such and have little to do with charges of bioconservatism.

Just as other feminists have criticized the vision of the human as autonomous or a carrier of pure rationality, I criticize transhumanism because it turns the boundless rationality once thought to conquer nature back upon human beings to remake them in accordance with this rational image. In this way, rather than going beyond the notion of an autonomous rational subject, transhumanism merely expands these ideals into a posthuman world. And what emerges from this world is not a hybrid that has no origin—as Haraway envisioned—a being outside of hierarchies that privilege men over women and culture over nature, including the human/animal, organism/machine, and physical/non-physical divides, putting stigmatizing norms into question (Haraway 1991, 151–153). Instead, transhumanists envision an extension of capabilities further into space and time and the multiplication and maximization of autonomy and intellect. Transhumanism is the realization of these hierarchical privileges, now extended. Transhumanism's imagined "cyborg" does not celebrate difference but rather the maximization and optimization of familiar valued traits such as cognitive ability and rational choice. These valued traits, transformed into ideals for the future, inform and support existing hierarchies that harm those who are believed to lack them.

TRANSHUMANIST STRATEGIES AND RHETORIC

But how and in what sense is the transhumanist goal of achieving posthumanism to be secured, according to transhumanists? I call attention to two primary enhancement strategies: first, the transcendence of embodiment (suggested by Bostrom) and, second, selection against stigmatized and unwanted traits associated with disability (suggested by Julian Savulescu). These strategies emphasize the rejection of embodiment as fragile and risky, facts which make Bostrom and Savulescu's work of special interest for feminist disability scholars, who seek to embrace these features of embodiment as part of an alternative ethic of vulnerability. I will attend to Bostrom and Savulescu's strategies for the remainder of this chapter.

I turn first to Bostrom. As we have seen, Bostrom's transhumanism is informed by the strong desire and the moral urgency of the avoidance of human suffering, especially suffering connected to disease and death (Bostrom 2003 and 2005a). He thus flags pursuit of posthumanism as a moral obligation, inspired by the sense that death is unjust and society is culpable for failing to address its victims (for echoes of this view see Harris 2011 and Savulescu 2001). Bostrom writes: "What is Guilt in Utopia? Guilt is our knowledge that we could have created Utopia sooner" (2010, 8 and 7). Bostrom's transhumanism is a fantasy of wish fulfillment, especially insofar as he focuses on the promise of immortality or decelerated aging.

When we consider Bostrom's fable of the dragon-tyrant, we should notice the ideological struggle in the city in particular. Who objects to the desire of the transhumanist to defeat death, aging, and the illnesses which are tied to them? The objector is those who preserve the status quo—the mayor, the one who is complacent (2005a). This fits with Bostrom's indictment of bioethics as rife with "status quo bias" (Bostrom and Ord 2006; cf. Agar 2010). But, I argue that a better interpretation of the "enemy" of transhumanism is the vulnerability of the body to mortality, which—if it is not rejected or ameliorated—will stymie the plan of enhancement for transhumanists. The dragon, representing death, inspires in transhumanists the need to defend the body through fundamental transformation. The fleshly human body becomes the transhumanist target of innovation as a result of its unacceptable vulnerability to injury and death.

Along these lines, Bostrom describes human bodies as fragile houses unfit for bliss and happiness: "it is not well to live in a self-combusting paper hut! . . . one day you or your children should have a secure home. Research, build, redouble your effort!" (2010, 2 and 5). Bostrom, here, is treating bodies as an enemy as if they belong to no one and weaves a fantasy of a disembodied intellect in search of a better location from which it can operate and experience life. This intellect, trapped in the body, appears to be the real posthuman who is waiting to be released. To reiterate, Bostrom rejects the human body as vulnerable and issues a moral imperative (echoed, as we shall see, in the work of Savulescu) to provide new sorts of bodies for one's children without vulnerability. Bostrom explicitly denigrates embodiment and, implicitly, dependence as part of his program of human enhancement. It is clear that Bostrom views mastery over the body, and, eventually, transcendence of embodiment as integral parts of the journey to a better, more moral and politically just future.

Bostrom's division of intellect from the body, and his suggestion of the possibility of intellectual release from the body through technology like mind uploading, supports entrenched hierarchies between body and mind. These hierarchies serve as rationales for devaluing persons with disabilities, especially cognitive disabilities. Relatedly, as we have seen, Bostrom commits transhumanism to an "emphasis on individual liberties," which casts humans in an atomistic light and downplays or devalues human interdependence (Bostrom 2005b, 4). Atomistic conceptions of the human also tend to devalue the lives of those with disabilities on the basis of the undesirability of dependence. These features of his account, together with his portrait of embodiment as risky, are troubling from a disability rights perspective; they suggest that we should avoid and eschew dependence, wherever it appears.

I turn now to the work of Julian Savulescu, editor-in-chief of the *Journal of Medical Ethics* and director of the Oxford Uehiro Centre for Practical Ethics. Savulescu's work, like Bostrom's, is motivated by moral urgency; Savulescu and Ingmar Persson claim that humans must enhance themselves morally or face extinction because of moral ineptitude. They draw on evolutionary psychology to describe "common-sense" morality and believe that this morality must be changed to mitigate or eliminate threats such as climate change and war (Savulescu 2009; Persson and Savulescu 2010 and 2012). Savulescu argues that "eugenic" genetic selection is the best way to achieve human enhancement (with Hemsley *et al.* 2006). Savulescu calls the obligation to select against certain traits "procreative beneficence" (2001, 425; cf. Savulescu 2002) and he makes clear that genetic markers for known disabilities are among the traits targeted as worse and to be avoided by those who are morally conscientious (Savulescu 2008). He believes that any trait which potentially curtails quality of life makes an embryo undesirable. Parents are morally responsible to choose future children on the basis of genetic testing in order to secure greater happiness and freedom for them—or at least provide the best chances at happiness and freedom (2001).

For Savulescu, in other words, parents have a moral obligation when reproducing to select for the traits that will contribute to the best chances for the best life (2001). Given existing technology, this means employing either selective abortion on the basis of the presence of certain traits uncovered via prenatal diagnosis or utilizing a combination of in-vitro fertilization and pre-implantation genetic diagnosis to select a favored embryo. Savulescu argues that the latter method is psychologically preferable for reproducers, although either is acceptable when following procreative beneficence (2001, 416). In the future, procreative beneficence would mean the moral imperative to use any technology available when reproducing to ensure the birth of the child with the best chances at the best life (cf. Savulescu and Kahane 2009).

Savulescu likens the reasoning involved in selecting embryos to playing the Wheel of Fortune; no matter how weak the link between genotype and expected eventual quality of life, he believes that a parent should select the embryo, of available embryos, with the best traits (2001, 414). He wants parents to play a game of chance—that is, to take a chance on choice. This applies, for instance, to cognitive ability, which he argues is essential to living a good life on most major versions of moral living (420). According to Savulescu, most moral conceptions of how to live a good life are based in or could be improved with maximized cognition (419–420). But, it also applies to myriad other traits, including traits for asthma and bad tempers, which could also affect quality of life (417 and 420). In Chapter 4, I discuss procreative beneficence and critique it using a version of Adrienne Asch's disability critique of genetic selection. There, I argue that procreative beneficence is ableist, sexist in its disregard for women who would be required to use it, and stigmatizes disabled and otherwise marked bodies.

Savulescu's focus on eliminating undesirable traits biologically obscures the ways these traits have come to be considered undesirable. With regard to disability specifically, his focus also obscures the way in which disability involves a lack of fit to the social world, which is malleable, or is socially constructed by way of stigma. His principle of procreative beneficence naturalizes disability and suggests that making the body malleable according to the dictates of the social is more important than the political goal of achieving accessibility for a variety of bodies and minds. Disability, viewed through procreative beneficence, is reduced to a genetic feature or prenatally visible trait which can be screened out or turned off by way of reproductive decision-making. Savulescu is thus performing a biological reduction reminiscent of the disputed "medical model" of disability, which would pose disability as purely biological. I return to these issues in the next chapter and defend an alternative model of disability.

The visible features of the fetus are limited to genetic anomalies and encourage the creation of classes among fetuses, arrayed along a range of normality that corresponds roughly to the traits we tolerate among already-existing persons,[8] already classed according to normalcy and, in many cases, heavily stigmatized (cf. Carlson 2002, 207–209). An example of such a class is persons with Down syndrome, whose prenatal prototype is selected against after detection of genetic markers in the fetus at rates over 90 percent in the United States (James 2009). By way of genetic profiles and diagnoses, a link is forged between a fetus and the features of those in existing communities that are not valued; thus, the potential child is deemed not desirable. Further, bias against already-existing persons is entrenched through this practice. According to Savulescu's principle of procreative beneficence, such a pregnancy should be ended or avoided as a matter of moral obligation. Unlike the gender disparity that might become a new factor in reproductive decision-making as the result of sex selection, it seems that there are no emergent reasons to curb this type of selection.

Using a critical disability lens to view procreative beneficence helps uncover the tableau of statistical risk and biopolitical logic embedded in Savulescu's account. For example, prenatal diagnostics presents medical, hereditary, and age-related statistics along with *risk* of deviation and associated costs to potential parents; it also requires decisive action in response to those statistics (see Waldschmidt 2005, 205). Parents can, using prenatal diagnostics, choose against "misfortune" by utilizing the platform of "statistical calculation" (204–205). As Savulescu puts it, reproduction becomes a game of the Wheel of Fortune, and potential parents must bet on the best embryo. In the case of an already-initiated pregnancy, meanwhile, parents would be urged to ask: do this potential child's chances justify continued pregnancy? Potential parents are thus asked to participate in the avoidance of risk to the population, and risk is most often figured as the risk of disability. Failure to manage risk is linked to disability. One must organize, select, and classify in order to best manage risk, and failure to do so is irresponsible. Savulescu's account of procreative beneficence encourages a disciplinary power in the clinic that buttresses the operation of biopolitics. Recall that biopolitics is comprised of both disciplinary and regulatory power, which mediate between individuals and the population in an attempt to ensure the health and homeostasis of the population as a whole.

Savulescu, in seeking a better future, suggests genetic selection as a primary enhancement strategy. In other words, we must engage in a practice of organizing, ranking, and eliminating potential persons from the population, if we are to survive. But, his account of the moral use of reproductive technology naturalizes disability traits and links risk and disability; in other words, it creates false chains of equivalences (disability is this body and, therefore, this body is risk). Bostrom's identification of vulnerability-as-enemy is echoed in Savulescu's contention that enhancement is necessary to stave off extinction and negative genetic selection will achieve enhancement. As exemplified in the work of Bostrom and Savulescu, transhumanism views the human body as bad because it is seen through the lens of risk, especially the risk of disablement, and views biotechnology as good because it enables choice.

For the transhumanist, positive and negative eugenics are linked together. Transhumanism repeatedly treats the two as co-extensive: to rid the world of disability *is* to enhance the human being—enhancement seems to require the rejection of disability and embodiment as risk and limitation. The logic of biopolitics, according to Foucault, establishes the following principle: "the very fact that you let more die will allow you to live more" (2003b, 255). Thomas Lemke biopolitics as placing "the health of one person in a direct relationship with the disappearance of another" (2011, 42). Here, Foucault and Lemke are pointing to racism as the element within biopolitics that allows the expression of sovereign power—that is, within a politics of life, racism gives power space to kill. As I argued in the Introduction, a robust understanding of how disability is deployed in bioethical contexts should be layered on to racism's function in biopolitics, so that we can understand disability as a primary location of power's negative expression.

Admittedly, transhumanists believe all human bodies are wanting and should be enhanced. Common human capabilities are not, for transhumanists, the endpoint of human progress but a shaky beginning. Transhumanists reject Norman Daniels' normative concept of species-typical functioning, as many disability rights activists and theorists have done. At least at first, then, it seems that transhumanists do *not* value the disabled body less than the abled body; rather, they consider all bodies to be in some sense deficient. This would be an improvement upon the view that the species-typical body is acceptable while bodies that deviate are not. But, it recalls Foucault's contention that biopower interprets threats differently from traditional sovereign power: in biopolitical contexts, "death was no longer something that suddenly swooped down on life—as in an epidemic. Death was now something permanent, something that slips into life, perpetually gnaws at it, diminishes it and weakens it" (Foucault 2003b, 244). We must be constantly vigilant against the threat of diminishment and this threat is mobile, attaching here or there according to biopolitical logic of culling from the inside.

Further, transhumanism explicitly rejects the disabled body and can increase stigma against persons with disabilities in two ways. First, it plays upon fears of disablement. As I have shown and will continue to demonstrate, transhumanist thinkers emphasize the fragility of the body and its susceptibility to *risk*. Taking Bostrom's image of the body as a paper hut together with Savulescu's focus on prenatal or preimplantation genetic profiles—which make the fetus a site of statistical risk—the risk of refusing transhumanist aims appears as the risk of disablement. This makes a disabled body the symbol of a feared outcome and a stand-in for death. Instead of seeing disability as a complex interrelationship between the body, social structures, and social norms, disability becomes the outcome of a too-complacent posture toward death and "technophobia." Second, the transhumanist point of view endorses a hierarchy of value and well-being among lives on the basis of capabilities; that is, the *greater the number* of capabilities, the larger the opportunity range, the better the life. Disability theorists, contra transhumanists, have worked to disentangle well-being from capability and argue that while capability is valuable, the lack of a capability should not be assumed to diminish well-being (e.g. Asch 2003, 318). So, disability is a special subject of concern for transhumanism as they work to classify, organize, and expel the abnormal from the population. I pick up this thread again in Chapter 4, where I claim that there is a deep divide between transhumanism and disability rights projects.

Bostrom combines Kant's motto, which exhorts readers to have courage to use intelligence, with Bacon's imperative of mastery, and thereby encourages seeking mastery over the body. The body also appears as an impediment to autonomy, making mastery of the body even more essential (Hauskeller 2012, 43). The division between intellect and body, and the possibility of intellectual release from the body through technology, recalls old hierarchies between body and mind. These hierarchies have served and can still serve as rationales for devaluing persons with disabilities, especially intellectual disability. Relatedly, Bostrom commits transhumanism to an "emphasis on individual liberties," which casts humans in an atomistic light and downplays or devalues human interdependence (Bostrom 2005b, 4). Atomistic conceptions of the human are also targets for disability theory, as they tend to devalue the lives of those with disabilities. Transhumanist visions seek to curtail or eliminate dependence and vulnerability rather than embracing these features as shared or as a starting point for ethics.

CONCLUSION

Transhumanist calls for the use of science and technology to make life better feed off common fears of death and pain, and cause us to frantically act in order to attempt to stave off both. Transhumanism is appealing because it promises wish fulfillment, but in our attempts to arrange future populations to reflect utopian wishes we twist the screw for already-existing, vulnerable persons and subject them to practices of classification and exclusion. Nick Bostrom advocates for the pursuit of posthumanity by way of the following argument:

> [Consider] our current ignorance and the vastness of the as-yet unexplored terrain. Let S_h be the 'space' of possible modes of being that could be instantiated by someone with current human capacities. Let S_p be the space of possible modes of being that could be instantiated by someone with posthuman capacities. In an intuitive sense, S_p is enormously much larger than S_h. (2008, 122)

This argument begs the question regarding the desirability of enhancement and one is cornered; bigger is always better and better is always better. Bostrom builds a specific vision of the future by way of contrast, without justifying why his means—intervention upon the body—are the appropriate path to get to that future. Further, the future he desires remains unknowable, despite his assurances that it will cohere with current human values. He invokes the idea of unknowability of that future when he writes, in the voice of a posthuman: "You could say that I feel surpassing bliss. But, these are words invented to describe human experience. What I feel is as far beyond human feeling as my thoughts are beyond human thought" (2005b, 3).

Transhumanism requires action to bring about desired futures and makes appeals for social investments, which often require misrepresentations of the present and exaggeration of hopes for the future. Some bioethicists have suggested enhancement is one way to achieve long-standing goals, like reducing negative environmental impacts, because it has the potential power (if we pursue it) to create human beings who are more sociable (less selfish and more altruistic) in their dealings (Liao *et al.* 2012). Transhumanists, in an amplification of this move, argue that enhancement is a strong moral imperative since it can create humans who have greater moral aptitude, which we need to do for fear that we will become extinct (Persson and Savulescu 2010 and 2012, Savulescu 2009). Transhumanist ideals include wide access to technology, in part in order to address frequent concerns that (expensive) enhancement technology will only be available to the lucky few, making entrenched inequality even more permanent (Bostrom 2009; Fukuyama 2004). Yet, such wide access is unlikely and dependent, as Bostrom appears to admit, on a better and a more global democracy than those currently enjoyed.

Transhumanist utopias are Romantic *human* dreams. Especially in Bostrom's work, transhumanists emphasize romantic feelings of happiness, even-temperedness, relief from suffering, and "zest"—all of which are understood as a *result* of choosing one's future. In other words, choice-making unlocks bliss. Bostrom writes of physical and mental changes which will accompany a chosen transhumanist future: "You begin to treasure almost every moment of life; you go about your business with zest; and you feel a deeper warmth and affection for those you love, but you can still be upset and even angry on occasions where upset or anger is truly justified and constructive" (2008, 111). Bostrom also describes increased kindness to animals, better political efforts (more justice), and better ecological support. Finally, also recall that posthuman pleasures embedded in transhumanist futures are most often hyper-realized human *desires*, as in Bostrom's "Why I Want to be a Posthuman When I Grow Up," where he suggests that posthumans will enjoy intensely pleasurable music, friendships, and multiplayer games (2008). Bostrom again invokes the unknown, a realm of complete transcendence:

> As we seek to peer farther into posthumanity, our ability to concretely imagine what it might be like trails off. If, aside from extended healthspans, the essence of posthumanity is to be able to have thoughts and experiences that we cannot readily think or experience with our current capacities, then it is not surprising that our ability to imagine what posthuman life might be like is very limited. (2008, 112)
>
> . . .what you had in your best moment is not close to what I have now—a beckoning scintilla at most. If the distance between base and apex for you is eight kilometers, then to reach my dwellings requires a million light-year ascent. The altitude is outside moon and planets and all the stars your eyes can see. Beyond dreams. Beyond imagination. (2010, 3)

Michael Hauskeller rightly points out that for utopian transhumanists, the body is seen as a constraint, not merely a site, for action. For transhumanists: "[bodies] seem to prevent us from being entirely autonomous" (2012, 43). This, then, is especially true of bodies that are considered needy—that is, disabled bodies. I return to the pervasive transhumanist idea of bodily enhancement or disposal as a mode of multiplying choice and creating freedom throughout this project.

Examining these transhumanist arguments is a way to wonder about the good of enhancement and its maximizations and call into question the connection of atomized choice-making with happiness and bliss. Why is more strength, more intelligence, or a longer life good for us? In what sense is it better? What can "better," or even "best" mean? Why does enhancement thinking view freedom as the freedom to make choices, and, as I will detail in the next chapter, see un-enhanced bodies as impediments to this freedom?

Bioethicist John Harris would scoff at these questions—for him, enhancements are always about making one better, and better is always good. Transhumanist Julian Savulescu, giving too much credence to the quantitative over the qualitative, assumes simply that "better" at least means more intelligent, as measured by any available cognitive tests (2001, 414). But, the transhumanist vision of better *relies on what society now values;* indeed, as we have seen, Bostrom sees this as a point in its favor, as transhumanism therefore does not require investment in new, posthuman values to build a bridge from past to future (2012, 622). But, I read transhumanism as fundamentally informed by deep-seated prejudices concerning what bodies and lives are best. If conceptions of "better" do not question existing stigmas, they will reify them.

NOTES

1. This organization is now known as Humanity+, and Bostrom is no longer officially affiliated with it. James Hughes and Anders Sandberg, whose work is also explored here, are listed on the organization website as advisors to Humanity+ (http://humanityplus.org/).

2. CRISPR (clustered regularly interspaced short palindromic repeats) is one of three gene-editing procedures, which also include TALEN (transcription activator-like effector nucleases) and zinc fingers. TALEN and zinc fingers use proteins as scissors, but CRISPR uses nucleic acids to edit genes. TALEN was successfully used to treat a young leukemia patient in London in 2015 (Begley 2015). CRISPR is considered most promising, but experts have recommended it not be used for germline editing until the process is better developed (Baltimore *et al.* 2015).

3. For a full discussion of the playing God objection, see Coady 2011.

4. Katherine Hayles, a proponent of her own version of posthumanism, critiqued transhumanist Hans Moravec because of his dreams of extended autonomy. She writes: "When Moravec imagines 'you' choosing to download yourself into a computer, thereby obtaining through technological mastery the ultimate privilege of immortality, he is not abandoning the autonomous liberal subject but is expanding its prerogatives into the realm of the posthuman" (Hayles 1999, 287; cf. Wolfe 2009, xv).

5. "The impossibility [of imagining posthuman capacities] is more like the impossibility for us to visualize a twenty-dimensional hypersphere or to read, with perfect recollection and understanding, every book in the Library of Congress. Our own current mode of being, therefore, spans but a minute subspace of what is possible or permitted by the physical constraints of the universe. It is not farfetched to suppose that there are parts of this larger space that represent extremely valuable ways of living, feeling, and thinking" (Bostrom 2012, 106).

6. According to Bostrom, mind uploading "would involve first freezing a brain, then slicing it, then scanning the slices with some high-resolution scanning technique, then using automated image processing software to reconstruct and tag a very detailed 3d map of the original brain. The map would show all the neurons, the matrix of their synaptic interconnections, the strengths of these connections, and other relevant detail. Using computational models of how these basic elements operate, the whole brain could then be emulated on a sufficiently capacious computer" (2004, n. 6).

7. A positional good is a good that is only valuable if it is unequally distributed.

8. As I note in the Introduction, I do not mean this phrase to refer to embryos or fetuses. Rather, I mean to refer to adults and children with disabilities or conditions resonant with what we tend to think of as disability.

Chapter 2

Rethinking Disability

Dodging Definitions, Muddying Models

In this chapter, I consider competing models of disability. I take the transhumanist fantasy to be centered upon a chosen subject that is opposed to the risky disabled subject, so it is important to establish how this cleavage comes about, who the disabled subject is, and what I mean when I talk about disabilities. I use a *cultural model* of disability and the concept of *stigma* to navigate these issues. I move to support the claim I made in the Introduction that disabilities are socially constructed and culturally circumscribed. This leads to the conclusion that those marked as disabled are subject to systematic exclusions on the basis of that marking, not on the basis of fundamental features of their biology that can be overcome via technology.

While disability communities are sometimes treated as political minorities, like other groups that have sought civil rights and equal treatment, it is important to avoid the ways that a pervasive "minority model" might contribute to the marginalization of persons with disabilities and positions them as a *competing* group that participates in policing the border between disability and ability. In what follows, I discuss this and other issues in order to explore the consequences of different ways of thinking "disabilities" and their construction. This discussion will frame my analyses in Chapter 3 of the history of enhancement enthusiasm and in Chapter 4 of genetic selection as a key strategy for enhancement.

The background for this chapter lies in a Foucauldian understanding of the subject as socially constructed and teetering upon cleavages between the abnormal and normal. Foucault's explorations of abnormality inform multiple threads of investigation for him and appear throughout many of his works. Before I begin my work in this chapter, I turn to his early book *Discipline and Punish* and his later lecture series *Abnormal* to describe what Foucault means when he uses the term.

FOUCAULT AND THE CONSTRUCTION OF THE ABNORMAL SUBJECT

In a reflection upon his early work, Foucault writes: "I have tried to show how we have indirectly constituted ourselves through the exclusion of some others: criminals, mad people, and so on" (*Technologies* 146). This indirect constitution is a matter of classification and exclusion according to various discourse of knowledge, including, for example, criminal science and diagnosis. Foucault's interest in knowledge production, and therefore the operations of power, led him to investigate discourses—anything written, said, or communicated using signs—and institutions—mental hospitals, prisons, factors, schools, courts of law. These are places where people are put in the position to witness, judge, submit, defend, confess, and therefore engage in activities while enacting exact roles, categorized and organized according to the function of power and knowledge. So, Foucault investigates power and knowledge by looking at their minute effects in specific times and places on specific people. Power, then, is not a simple matter of a dyadic relationship between two persons, A and B, in which A is powerful and B, because she is influenced by A, experiences domination. For Foucault, power is a matter of networks of subjects and objects, is non-agential, and has both "negative" (what one might call constraining) and "positive" effects (what one might call self-expression). We build and engage our subjectivity in and through power. Specifically, as I have argued, bioethics discourse is embedded in a power regime that Foucault refers to as biopolitical.

Careful and context-specific historical investigation will provide us with key information with regard to the construction of subjectivity. If we follow Foucault's shift to discourses and institutions, we can begin to understand how people are regulated, disciplined, and produced by social forces. We can also see how the self-expression of one's subjectivity is conditioned by external systems. *Discipline and Punish* (1979) is one piece of Foucault's project. There, he tells a genealogical story regarding how punishment and control have changed over time, moving from the punishment of the body to the discipline of the subject, and describes the minute effects of different systems of punishment and control on subjectivity. Ultimately, the genealogy Foucault builds in *Discipline and Punish* is a genealogy of political technology and investigates the ancestry of the contemporary biopolitical state.

The initial moments of *Discipline and Punish* are taken up in a gruesome description of the lethal punishment in France of an attempted regicide, Robert-François Damiens, who was drawn and quartered in 1757 in front of the public in a wild display of state power. While this display was intense, it is also inefficient; the people might revolt upon seeing the naked display of power, and the operation of power requires the physical restraint of the object of punishment, Damiens. Public executions are an early political technology, now superseded. In contrast, through surveillance—a key ingredient of biopower—everyone is given a place. All subjects are conditioned as either normal or abnormal, and slotted into various fractured spaces, including hospitals, prisons, nursing homes, and in exile.

Foucault traces two examples within the development of the surveillance technique: the management of the plague and the exile of the leper (1979). The plague represents the ultimate disorder—in order to deal with the contagion, local governments improvised ways to impose order which required high investment (sentries who would manage quarantine) and hands-on surveillance (1979, 195–198). The second narrative is that of the leper, who is "marked" and excluded (198). Through exile, the leper is removed from the city and marked as abnormal. They are both classified and removed. The modern political technology of panoptic surveillance, discussed in the Introduction, inherits and recombines these strategies in ever-new ways; modern systems of control combine the strategy of containing the plague with the strategy of excluding the leper (199–200).

In *Abnormal* (2003a), Foucault describes how the abnormal criminal subject was produced, and thereby slated for surveillance, in the mid-twentieth century French courtroom. Penal discourses established a kind of truth, pulling from pseudoscience and folk psychology, by which matters of life and death can be decided. Psychiatric experts are asked to be witnesses with regard to the criminal's tendencies, providing a criminal prehistory in which characteristics are naturalized and made punishable: "After all, if he has stolen, it is basically because he is a thief" (2003a, 16).[1] In this way, the abnormal subject takes root. Taking this as a larger pattern, we can see the workings of biopolitics, the eye of which is trained upon the "species body" and supervises the "propagation births and mortality, the level of health, life expectancy and longevity, with all the conditions that can cause these to vary" (Foucault 1990, 139). These supervisions produce abnormal and normal subjectivities and are behind monstrous figures of all kinds which are subject to classification and exclusion.

Again, Foucault's understanding of the construction of the subject, in both its positive and negative inflections, provides a backdrop for my work in this chapter. Disability is historically, materially, and discursively connected to the idea of abnormality, and the idea of the disabled subject—which individual persons engage and reject, build upon and critique—is produced, not born.

THINKING DISABILITY

I turn now to explore and analyze some of the many meanings of disability. An analysis of Dena Davis' work on genetic counseling, particularly *Genetic*

Dilemmas, can motivate the problem of defining disability in bioethics (2010). In it, she slips between different ways of conceiving disability in a way that will help us get clear on what some of the main difficulties are in conceiving disability.

Davis argues that harm results when disabilities are genetically chosen by parents; specifically, a future harm of narrowed possibilities, a closing-off of the so-called right to an open future (2010, 59–60; 1997, 14). But, she also seems to peg harm as an endemic element of her definition of disability, especially when she talks about her primary case study: deafness. For instance, as a response to the Deaf community's self-identification as a cultural minority, Davis writes: "On the other side of the argument is the evidence that deafness is a very serious disability. Deaf people have incomes thirty to forty percent below the national average. The state of education for the deaf is unacceptable by anyone's standards; the typical deaf student graduates from high school unable to read a newspaper" (1997, 12–13). But, how are these statistics *evidence* of disability? Given a context in which most deaf students are not provided with an interpreter in the classroom,[2] it seems that the statistics Davis lays out here are merely evidence of prejudice and stigma against certain modes of embodiment and do not signal something inherent one might call "disability." We could parallel these statistics with statistics regarding, for example, the low-income status or imprisonment rates of racial and ethnic minorities—these numbers are evidence of prejudice, not direct results of features such as the color of one's skin, one's lineage, or one's birthplace. Similarly, it is not the fact of deafness that leads to the educational difficulties Davis mentions; instead, it is a lack of accommodation. Also, note that Davis is opposing "cultural minority" with "disability"—she assumes that the two concepts cannot overlap, without interrogating them.

Another example of the way Davis shifts among notions of disability is apparent in the following passage: "Ethically, we would certainly include destroying someone's hearing as being a '*harm*'; legally, one would undoubtedly receive compensation if one were rendered deaf due to someone else's negligence. Many deaf people, however, have recently been arguing that deafness is not a *disability* at all, but a linguistic and cultural identity" (2010, 65, emphasis mine, cf. Lane 2010). So, if deafness is not a disability for the Deaf community, Davis seems to be saying, they would not consider it harmful—therefore, disability and harm are employed here as one and the same thing.

Finally, Davis considers the famous Gallaudet University movement in 1988, when University students and faculty demanded a Deaf president for Gallaudet, protesting the appointment of a hearing president made by the board of trustees (The "Deaf President Now" campaign). Of it, she writes: "Looking at photographs taken during those tumultuous weeks, it is clear that the Gallaudet students regarded themselves as one more oppressed minority, not as a disabled group" (2010, 65). Here, Davis opposes the concepts of "oppressed minority" and "disabled group" as if it were impossible for one collective to be both at the same time. This is another slippage: if Davis believes these two ways of describing a group are mutually exclusive, she fails to make her reasons explicit.

Because Davis focuses on Deaf culture, it is important to note that Davis is correct when she asserts that "many deaf people, however, have recently been arguing that deafness is a not a *disability* at all, but a linguistic and cultural identity" (2010, 65). In other words, at least some deaf persons, who identify as part of the Deaf community, reject the label of disability. The questions we are left with include: what is disability? Is it embodied "harm?" Does it make protest impossible? If disability culture exists, does that make it necessary to shed the label of "disability," as some in the Deaf community and Davis seem to believe? Why does identifying as "disabled" seem to eclipse and delimit other identities which a person might take up?

Defining disability and working with disability as a political identity is a difficult task because current and historical prejudice must be taken into account (Parens and Asch 2000, 5). For many in the disability rights community, "discrimination results when people in one group fail to imagine that people in some 'other' group lead lives as rich and complex as their own" (8). Disabled academic and activist William J. Peace has argued that the current euthanasia debate, which tends to assume that death is preferable to living a life with disability, expresses this failure of the imagination (2012). Surely, however, as Peace also argues, dismal institutional failures and a lack of social responsiveness are also to blame and can be the ultimate sources for imaginative failures (2013a, 2013b). At the very least, it is clear that the notion of disability is fraught with value judgments and subject to deep stigma and multiple exclusions. To call someone disabled involves an evaluative judgment as well as a description. Imported into the concept are complex and shifting stereotypes that are difficult to reverse. And, illness and limitations connected to disabilities makes politically ironic "reversal" moves open to other groups, like people of color, much harder to accomplish. Disability theorist Irving Zola writes of the problem: "Could [disability activists] yell, 'Long live cancer' 'Up with multiple sclerosis' 'I'm glad I had polio!' 'Don't you wish you were blind?'" (1993, 168).

Further, isolation issues among persons with disabilities make it difficult for individuals to organize together. A person may be integrated with family or friends who may not and likely do not share their disability, and so, writes Zola, "they are socialized into the world of the 'normal' with all its values, prejudices and vocabulary" (1993, 167). This particular kind of isolation is largely unique to the case of disability, although others—including those who identify or are identified with excluded sexual identities—will share in the problem of isolation.[3] Further, isolation goes beyond these issues to systematized social practices of isolation like "special" (usually segregated) education, warehousing in nursing homes (even for children), and sheltered workshops which are legally permitted to pay persons with disabilities subminimum wage. Uneven allegiance to disability identities among persons whose embodiment or experiences might fall under relevant categories contributes to the complications of related *political* questions of disability identity. Disability theorist James Charlton discusses the psychic alienation incurred by social alienation and stigma, which can in turn bar persons with disabilities from claiming disability identity (2010).

Another difficulty is that if disability as a phenomenon at least somehow begins with or incorporates traits borne by the body, there are no uncontested frameworks for which traits *count* as disabilities—what about mental illness and alcoholism? Furthermore, many tend to think of disabilities as existing along a spectrum from more to less serious or debilitating, an inherited tendency of looking at disability through a medical lens. So, layered on top of the difficulty of saying whether someone with diabetes, for example, has a disability, we also encounter the difficulty of describing which, among a variety of forms of embodiment, are considered "serious" disabilities. And, of course, professionals with power to impact the shape of discourse, like genetic counselors, policymakers, and medical and educational professionals, cannot agree. The very act of creating or discursively supporting spectrums and taxonomies shapes the contours of disability, creating gradations of stigma and a variety of political and social responses.

Importantly for the discussion in this book, bioethicists Erik Parens and Adrienne Asch demonstrate that "genetics professionals have very different ideas of what is and what is not" a trait that is significantly disabling (2000, 9, cf. 261). Specific examples of contested traits for geneticists include: "cleft lip/palate, neurofibromatosis, hereditary deafness, insulin-dependent diabetes, Huntington disease, cystic fibrosis, sickle cell anemia, Down syndrome, and manic depression"; these traits "were deemed serious by some professionals and not serious by others" (9). Designating a trait as serious signals that the trait should be medically intervened upon—that is, that it is in need of correction. And, of course, in addition to inherited traits, illness or accident can also be disabling; examples include blindness, deafness, paraplegia or limb loss, along with traumatic brain injury.

As for more thoroughgoing schemes, the World Health Organization (WHO) distinguishes among *impairment*, *disability* and *handicap*:

> Paralysis of the legs (perhaps resulting from polio or spina bifida) is the impairment; the inability to walk is the disability; but it is "the social consequences of that disability—the refusal of employers to hire a disabled person . . . that

> renders him or her handicapped." A disability becomes a handicap due to the choices of individuals and organizations. Handicaps are the result of social choices; they are not part of the "fabric of the moral universe." Because they are chosen, they can be changed. (Steinbock 2000, 113–114, quoting from Scheer and Groce 1998, 24)

It is clear from this tripartite scheme that some would agree that disability is both physical and social. In other words, perhaps we could tentatively say that collective political action can relieve a "handicap" through social measures, and medicine can relieve an "impairment," and both bear upon a person's potential or actual disability. Yet, from here, the issue only gets more complicated. Consider again the way that an impairment/handicap or impairment/disability distinction operates as an analog of the sex/gender distinction—are impairment and sex therefore "natural" categories that are not constructed symbolically or socially? Furthermore, schemes like this serve to deny or hide positive aspects of disability identity. How do the biological and the social interact, and in what sense does medicine play a role in the lives of persons with disabilities? Should medicine play this role? How does this identity actually operate? To begin to answer these questions in a serious way, we must turn to diverse work in disability theory.

I discuss the drawbacks and complicated reception each model has received among theorists. The theoretical models I discuss set out to accomplish very different things, and so I orient models of disability not only conceptually but also in terms of the goals and motivations for their construction. Taking a birds' eye view of models of disability in the pages that follow will help illuminate the way in which persons posed as "abled" and posed as "disabled" meet each other at the borders between these roles.[4]

MODELS OF DISABILITY

Models of disability tend to be posed as solutions to problems facing persons with disabilities or approximate what is found to be problematic about existing social, political, and cultural conditions. That is, models of disability are typically meant to either *symbolize* or *solve* problems of exclusion and stigma that come along with physical and mental difference. More rarely, methods are used to symbolize what it is like, experientially, to have a disability; for this, something like a phenomenological or materialist account is needed (for this type of work, see Iwakuma 2002; Scully 2008; I return to these more fluid schemes, below, by way of the "cultural model"). In disability studies, experiential accounts are also expressed through non-fictional, first-personal vignettes (e.g. Finger 2007), life writing (e.g. Mintz

2007), fiction (see the *Disability Rag*, now the *Ragged Edge*), and poetry (see Kuppers 2006 and *Ragged Edge*). Models of disability should be conceived of as Weberian ideal types, which will admit of variations and bordercrossings in theoretical work.

The Moral Model and the Charity Model

The "moral model" and the "charity model" are posed critically by disability theorists to persuade those who reflect on them to reject them as limiting and stigmatizing. Both also serve the higher purpose of telling a nuanced disability history and building an understanding of the social influences that form experiences of disabilities. The *moral model* appears in ancient theological texts such as the Bible, Koran and the Midrash (rabbinic reflections on and interpretations of the Talmud). On this model, disability of any sort can be understood as the result of sin—perhaps generational sin which is passed down from one's ancestors, or perhaps personal sin which has resulted in affliction from above (Goffman 1963, 1–2). Disability theorist Henri-Jacques Stiker writes: "This is illustrated in the Pharisees' question to Jesus concerning a blind man: 'Who sinned? Was it he or his family?'" (1999, 27). This model figures disability as impurity, attached to a person rendered therefore unfit to be in the presence of a higher power, and has been the basis for "ritual exclusion" in diverse religious contexts (Stiker 1999, 25).

The linkage between moral desert and disability has not disappeared with time. This is evidenced in the rhetorical question "What have I done to deserve this?" It also appears in popular entertainment, which regularly uses markers of physical and mental differences as a way to indicate moral inferiority or the beginning of an immoral career to audiences (e.g. The Joker and Two-Face in *The Dark Knight*; Al Pacino's iconic role as Tony Montana in *Scarface* and Ernst Blofeld in *You Only Live Twice*; cf. Zola 1993, 169). As Susan Sontag argues in her *Illness as Metaphor,* physical deformity and moral evil or criminality are linked together in the dominant cultural imaginary (1978–1989). Paul Longmore's essay "Screening Stereotypes: Images of Disabled People in Television and Motion Pictures" later expanded upon this claim (1987). Longmore pointed to the consistent tropes of disability which appear in television and film. Two of the most constant are the disabled "villain" like Doctor No, Doctor Strangelove, or Miguelito P. Loveless, and the disabled "monster" like Victor Hugo's "hunchback" or the eponymous Phantom of the *Phantom of the Opera* (1987, 67–68).[5] Disability theorists Sharon Snyder and David Mitchell develop a nuanced theoretical understanding of the use of disability as "prosthesis" for the movement of plots and as dramatic device in their work *Narrative Prosthesis: Disability and the Dependencies of Discourse* (2000).

The *charity model* is much newer if we use an ancient timeline, but also has deep historical roots that continue to reverberate today. This model critically assesses charity discourses, economies, and institutions, which construe disabled persons as objects of pity. Charity circumscribes characteristics that persons experiencing disability can exhibit and still receive benefits. These expectations, in turn, limit the opportunities of those with disabilities. Charity undergirds the Jerry Lewis telethon (funded by the Muscular Dystrophy Association and led by Lewis from 1966 to 2010), a practice that actor Lewis defended against objections from the Disability Rights Movement (DRM) which claim that the telethons and associated advertisements are degrading ("Jerry Lewis" 1991). This is especially problematic in light of the disabled characters Lewis has offensively portrayed. Lewis has been accused of infantilizing disability and obtaining income for his charity merely through generating pity among viewers, thereby frustrating the goals of disability rights activism (Stevenson, Harp, and Gernsbacher 2011). Lewis' defense of the telethons was bitter; he once shot back: "If you don't want to be pitied because you're a cripple, stay in your house" (Ervin 2009).

Snyder and Mitchell analyze the charity model in the nineteenth century and forward. For example, they investigate classical literature, such as Herman Melville's *The Confidence-Man: His Masquerade* (first published in 1857). They write:

> Charity organizations assured that "excessive" need could be met with stern disapproval, moral disapprobation, and patronizing religious instruction. At the same time charity also provided a public benefit in recognizing individual contribution as a sign of beneficence, generosity, and commitment to capitalist values of self-reliance. Charity's provision of such an outlet for moralistic example demonstrates what disability historian Paul Longmore defines as the practice of conspicuous contribution: a cultural ritual in which the "economically able" garishly donate in public venues to help disabled people and bolster their own renown. Within these economic rituals, "disability" itself becomes a matter of performative interdependency as disabled bodies are made to appear unduly dependent and donors further solidify their own social value as able benefactors. (2006, 41, quoting Longmore 1997, 146)

So, charity simultaneously sets up roles for the abled and roles for the disabled, and specifies an acceptable level of need for the disabled while also reinforcing capitalistic values that serve to define and oppose disability and ability in the first place—that is, roles related to production and consumption. And, the charity model provides a moral education for persons who are abled *by way of* the persons with disabilities and their bodies, the object of charity.

Charity still plays a primary role in providing basic goods and services to persons with disabilities, whose unemployment rates are astronomical and who are legally employable for less than minimum wage. Further, I find that, in theoretical work, the framing of a possible moral education for the abled *by way of* the disabled reappears. Philosopher Christie Hartley, who aims to show that the political and social inclusion of persons with disabilities is consistent with and required by justice (as justice is understood in core theories belonging to the social contract tradition in liberalism), positions people with disabilities as teaching those around them core liberal virtues. To accomplish her aim of including in a theory of justice those thought to lack the two moral powers outlined by John Rawls, Hartley argues that persons with disabilities make "substantial contributions" to their communities and explains that they are connected to the aim of creating, establishing, and maintaining a "society based on relations of mutual respect" with reciprocity as ruling norm. To discuss the cooperative contributions she has in mind, Hartley relates several primary narratives about persons with disabilities.

She details the relationship between philosopher Eva Feder Kittay and her daughter, Sesha, who, despite her constraints in the area of language, "communicates some of her preferences" and enjoys music, experiences which can be shared with others (2009, 151). Hartley also reports that Sesha provides Kittay with emotional support that Kittay estimates as invaluable. Hartley further mentions the relationship between philosopher Sophia Wong and her brother, Leo, who helps "the Wongs realize the importance of patience and compassion," when the family plays card games together (*ibid.*). Hartley writes: "By resisting the temptation to take advantage of him and go for a win, the members of Leo's family develop skills that are distinctive of *fair* cooperation" (*ibid.*). Hartley's good intentions are dissolved in these flat descriptions of rich relationships, which figure disabled persons as providing a moral (in this case also a political) education to those around them.

The moral and charity models were constructed by critics in order to say something about and protest historical or current treatment of persons with disabilities. In other words, to describe these models is to simultaneously protest their continued influence in the lives of those with disabilities. No part of either model is meant to isolate what disability "means" prescriptively or propose definitions of disability for the future.

The Medical Model

The *medical model* of disability is still supreme in mainstream culture but just as highly charged for disability theorists as the moral and charity models. The medical model of disability, on its strongest version, orients all descriptions and explanations of disability in biological particulars. Negative experiences encountered by a person with disability, including discomforts and lack of freedoms and capabilities, are all, on this model, due solely to disability's character as a biological issue—a problem of health, to be dealt with medically (Daniels, Rose, and Zide 2009, 75–76; Saxton 2000, 149). As opposed to the charity and moral models, the medical model does mean to prescriptively describe and define disability. What the World Health Organization described as "impairment" (e.g. paraplegia, polio, loss of vision) becomes, on this model, the entirety of the concept of disability. To put it more succinctly still, the medical model, broadly construed, defines disability as limitation located in or stemming from the body (Smith 2009). So, on the one hand, the medical model is constructed in earnest in order to analyze and consider the effects of disability.

Yet, on the other hand, what some consider an earnest model, that is, a model meant to describe what disability actually is, stimulates fervent critique and is considered by disability theorists the fountainhead of stigmatizing and marginalizing taxonomies, labels, and stereotypes. For disability rights activists, the medical model is "an inaccurate interpretation of disability forming the basis of oppressive and exploitative relationships between non-disabled and disabled people" (Smith 2009, 15). The medical model views individuals through the lens of their role as a "patient"—as if everyone who has experienced limitation or been stigmatized for a trait is, therefore, a permanent patient (Saxton 2000, 149). This framing causes unnecessary social isolation and unjust social treatment.

Thus, the medical model, in its treatment of disability as pathology and illness, contributes to the isolation and devaluation of persons with disabilities. As long as persons with disabilities are labeled "ill" and their identity as disabled is tied up in interactions with the medical establishment, they become part of a hidden minority which is accounted for statistically (Zola 1993, 168). The representation of disability through statistics leads to the circumscription of disability as a risk of embodiment.

The fact that mainstream discourse relies on medical understandings of disability also leads to pervasive institutional abuses, because the medical model makes the clinical institution the appropriate home for persons with disabilities. In 2012, federal officials sent Florida Attorney General Pam Bondi a letter on behalf of more than 200 children (including infants) who were living in nursing homes for (on average) three years; the regulators allege that the state is violating the Americans with Disabilities Act and the children's civil liberties by housing them there. Florida State University law professor Paolo Annino, along with other attorneys in Florida, filed a suit in corroboration with the letter sent to Bondi. They noted that more than 3,300 children would be rehoused in nursing homes because of state funding cuts eliminating the nursing services that would allow the children to remain at home. Nursing homes, meant to care for the aging, are ill-equipped to deal with the young and present significant blocks to maturation, relationship-building and sexual development—the result of basic institutional restraints on schedules and rooming (Kennedy 2012). According to the press,

> the suit and federal regulators say children languish in facilities, sharing common areas with elderly patients and having few interactions with others, rarely leaving the nursing homes or going outside. After visiting children in six nursing homes, investigators noted that children are not exposed to social, education and recreational activities that are critical to child development. Educational opportunities are limited to as little as 45 minutes per day. (Kennedy 2012)

Housing young children and infants in nursing homes is only intelligible through a medical model that considers disability a medical condition for which health services are the primary, or even only, concern. Because social sites for the responsive reception of persons with disabilities are sorely lacking, these individuals are marginalized and hidden by inappropriate placement in nursing homes. In impact, the move to institutionalize in nursing homes (as well as group homes, depending on the circumstances) serves the same purpose as "ugly laws" or "unsightly beggar ordinances" in California, Chicago, Columbus, Ohio, and Omaha, Nebraska. Chicago's turn of the century "ugly laws" made it illegal to be in public spaces with many disabilities (Schweik 2010). Social marginalization is socially constructed, and it is easy to devalue and dismiss groups that one cannot see.

Ironically, total institutions for persons with disabilities which presume that disabilities are medical issues create ill health. For example, there is a long institutional history of the denial of appropriate nutrition and desired meals to persons with disabilities. Food is regulated and used as punishment or reward in institutionalized settings. Jeff Moyer, a disability rights activist whose brother, Mark, was kept in a state-run mental institution in Ohio for 30 years, recorded a series of interviews with those whose relationship to food was defined in these contexts (a transcribed excerpt is available online via Moyer 2007). Caretakers evidently believed that a person's "bad" behavior could be mitigated by denying her food: [Woman's voice]: "People didn't receive meals, when they were 'misbehaving,' if you will. . ." [Woman's voice]: "If a staff person felt that, let's say, someone had misbehaved, they would just walk right up and say 'You're done' and take their meal, whether they were finished or not, they were done." Snacks were denied, and certain individuals were given only blended foods as part of a behavior program.

This situation made food a matter of desperation. [Woman's voice]: "Someone choked, because they had stolen food" (Moyer 2007). Food was not considered a means of nourishment for those living at the Ohio institution; instead, it was deployed as a means of behavioral control: [Man's voice]: "I don't know why, whether they took his food away from him also, or what, but he just, he was very malnourished, terribly so." Individuals living there were sometimes malnourished, because assisted eating was not provided or even considered: [Woman's voice]: "My husband and his mother came down the next day and found out, you know, that nobody seemed to know that she couldn't feed herself" (*ibid.*). This circumstance of neglect recalls Foucault's contention that biopower "fosters life or disallows it to the point of death" (Lemke 2011, 36).

The medical model cannot accept social factors playing a role in disablement, and so necessarily ignores the stigmatizing cultural and political construction. It conflates the prejudicial treatment experienced by persons with disabilities or simply their social experiences in general with traits of the body—it naturalizes them. For philosophers Kristjana Kristiansen, Simo Vehmas, and Tom Shakespeare, "the expression *medical model of disability* has become a common nickname for a one-sided view that attributes the cause of individual's deficits either to bad luck (accidents), to inadequate health practices (smoking, bad diet), or to genes" (2009, 2). The medical model, therefore, is a model which describes the causes of disability as individual, and divorced from social life, and is also a model which treats disability (even if disability has social aspects known to be negative) as naturalized and inevitable or the result of individual choices. It justifies isolation, neglect, and death. There is no one to blame but the body, unless of course, one also chooses to blame an individual's bad lifestyle and unhealthy decision-making. On this model, one can call disability "tragic" and yet evade responsibility for the tragedy of poor treatment (Smith 2009, 16).

Further, the medical model invites essentialism. Disability under this model is necessarily a "fixed" and "permanent" condition, which "inevitably causes 'dependency' between disabled and non-disabled people"; resulting dependency is likewise depicted as permanent (Smith 2009, 15; cf. Barnes 1991, 2). The medical model insists that disability cannot be separated from dependency, but under this model, dependency is a product of biology, not interpersonal relationships, and is necessarily negative. This runs against feminist insights that relationships and embodiment are fundamental parts of selfhood and therefore of autonomy (e.g. Meyers 2005). Further, differences between non-disabled and disabled persons are essentialized (Smith 2009, 16–17). Meanwhile, normality is also naturalized under this model (17). Ways in which cultural and society construct shifting meanings of normality, as revealed in my genealogy of enhancement thinking carried out in the next chapter, are hidden. These discursive conditions work together to naturalize and materialize disability.

The Social Model

The *social model*, also known as the British social model, first articulated by disability scholar and activist Michael Oliver in the early 1980s, is meant as a direct response to and rejection of the medical model. In that sense, it perhaps swings the pendulum back too far in the other direction, thus leaving itself open to inevitable revision. This model serves as a rallying cry and an effective political tool for disability rights movements and disability activists globally. Unlike the charity and moral models, it is not articulated in order to be rejected, or to illuminate the past; instead, it is future-oriented. That is because it describes disability primarily as originating in social failures with regard to *accommodation* for difference, and to describe it this way is to simultaneously require radical social change.

The social model posits that difficulties or differences in quality of life experienced by persons with disabilities are due to a lack of social accommodation rather than inherent qualities of the individual experiencing disability (Abberley 1987). Steven Smith calls a very common version of the social model the "politics of disablement" interpretation, in which "attention is directed . . . toward changing the social and political environment" (2009, 18). Here, a distinction is made between impairment and disability: "Impairment is associated with a particular medical condition, which may (or may not) lead to a disability" and "disability [is] associated with various social and political restrictions often (but not always) imposed upon people with impairments" (Smith 2009, 18). This distinction is in radical contrast to the medical model's conflation of impairment and disability, but fits with the WHO conceptual scheme. Importantly, many versions of the social model do *not* claim, as is sometimes supposed, that disabling traits are themselves neutral (Daniels, Rose and Zide 2009, 75). Rather, the more common claim is that regrettable aspects of disability *can be* neutralized as long as society understands and accommodates disability (Parens and Asch 2000, 24).

The social model improves upon the medical model in a number of obvious ways. It places new responsibilities on society to make room for physical and mental differences, and rejects the idea that one's body or "impairment" must necessarily lead to social and political restrictions. It points to the hidden ways that political and social decision-making directly cause or shape disability. It can demonstrate the infuriating irony of the "supercrip" trope, which poet, theorist and disability activist Eli Clare describes in his *Exile and Pride*, wherein Clare relates painful and difficult experiences of mountain-climbing as a person with cerebral palsy and the way his unsteady step takes him through rocky terrain (1999). These experiences, for Clare, unlock the door to the realization that he has internalized the supercrip imperative, which puts responsibility on the individual to overcome personal circumstances rather than placing responsibility for change and development squarely in political and social action.

But, the social model has devastating drawbacks which arise primarily from the framing of its rejection of the medical model. That is, in the social model's definition of any limitations connected to disability as merely social, a veil is thrown over the body and embodied first-person experiences, not describable in social or political terms, are obscured (Smith 2009, 18). It can invalidate pain, and serves to untether discussions about disability completely from the body. Further, impairment and disability are divided from each other, in an analogy with the distinction between sex and gender (Tremain 2006). In this way impairment is related to the body and disability is related to the social world. The distinction between impairment and disability treats impairment as immune to social construction.

The pervasiveness of the social model among disability activists has made it difficult to revise or abandon. For instance, Mairian Scott-Hill encounters the social model as a "new orthodoxy" (2004; cf. Kelly 2010).[6] Scott-Hill "proposes a postmodern, communicative paradigm which 'takes the view that social relations between people are necessarily complex'" (Kelly 2010, quoting from Scott-Hill 2004, 163). But, she experiences strong backlash; she claims that her view "tends to be interpreted by 'orthodox' social modellists as threatening the unity of disabled people's political campaigns and accused of promoting a relativistic world in which the 'fact' or 'reality' of disability can no longer be assured" (Scott-Hill 2004, 169). In other words, for some who promote the social model, if disability is seen as excessively fluid, political disability identity is threatened. This is a very undesirable standoff, especially since the social model is meant to capture the highly interpersonal and contextual nature of the politics of disablement.

But the social model opens important discussions and ushered in new activism, helping highlight accommodation and justice issues. It breaks free of the medical model's essentializing insistence that disabilities are biological facts. But, the distinction that the social model makes between impairment and disability leaves impairment itself a naturalized category, as if it is immune to social construction. And, it deprioritizes discussion of the body, pain, and limitation that feminist philosophers of disability, like Liz Crow, Liz French, and Jenny Morris, seek. According to disability theorists Shakespeare and Mark Erickson, these thinkers: "do not deny that society causes many problems, [but] they also feel that their bodies may cause difficulties, and they want any theory of disability to take account of the physical dimension to their lives" (Shakespeare and Erickson 2001, 195).

Most importantly, the social model frames disabilities as merely negative. On this model, "disability" conceptually marks a *failing* on the part of the social world and signals a *lack* of accommodation; when disability is discussed in this sense it falls into the trap of asserting that disability is inherently and also merely negative. For those in the disability rights movement, a movement often focused on the potential of persons with disabilities to be independent, this is not a good result. The social model, as an activist view, should be able to support the idea of disability as a banner and a positive identity that brings people together—disability should be more than simply a problem to be solved. But, if disability *is* social failure, and accommodation problems are overcome, does the concept of disability disappear, along with disability identities themselves? It appears that for the social model the answer is yes: the social model valorizes "ordinary citizenship" insofar as it takes accomplishing this type of citizenship for all as the aim of ameliorating lack of access in the social world (Smith 2009, 19; cf. Kelly 2010). In that sense, the social model will not represent a cultural critique of the complex relationship between norm and deviance, or negation or lack and social acceptance. Disability theorist Tanya Titchkosky writes:

> So common is it to map disability through a series of negations that it might be easy to miss the strangeness of such a process. This strangeness is revealed when we try to map others in a similar fashion, for example, a man is a person lacking a vagina. It would seem ridiculous today to conceive of gender in terms of negation. However, it is still common to regard the disabled body as a life constituted out of the negation of able-bodiedness and, thus, as nothing in and of itself. (2002, 103)

Although the negativity of disability is not equated to individual tragedy under the social model the way it is under the medical model, simply relocating the concept of disability from the body to the social is not enough. Mairian Scott-Hill (Corker) received backlash for her "postmodern" view of disability, which calls into question disability as concrete fact; yet, the social model should be called into question for its characterization of disability as a negative marker of social failure, while simultaneously failing to investigate the cultural constructs of deviance and disability.

The Minority Model

The *minority model* of disability overlaps tightly with the social model, but presents unique issues. Taking the social model's interpretation of disability as a basis, it primarily focuses on the attainment of civil rights (Dell Orto and Marinelli, 1995). But, unlike the social model, it seeks to neutralize the perceived negativity of impairment. This is accomplished, for instance, by claiming that wheelchair use is variation rather than limitation, and calling into question the normalcy of walking as a mode of mobility. The Deaf community takes up a variety of this model by way of its claim that deafness is a culture, not a disability. But, it is unclear why the label of disability or disability as an identity and minority claims related to culture must oppose one another—it seems that in order to make a "minority" claim, some believe that a "disability" identity must be shed or shifted elsewhere. I will use the example of the controversy surrounding "direct funding" in order to begin describing more concrete problems connected to the minority model.

Direct funding refers to a situation in which persons with disabilities receive government funds to "hire and sometimes train" service (care) providers and thus "manage their own personal assistance" by disbursing payments for their own care (Kelly 2010). This is a major goal of "personal assistance activism" and fits with a minority model scheme of disability. Personal assistance activism, however, puts to the side concerns about minimum wage, labor standards, and working conditions for those providing the care work. Because funds available to persons with disabilities are limited and often far too low, part of "personal assistance activism" will be the attempt to keep payments for care work as low as possible in order to manage one's budget. In other words, minority politics advocacy around "direct funding" pits persons with disabilities against care workers in a struggle over scarce resources. It places those with disabilities in a position of power over those workers who provide their care because little to no oversight is built in to the system (Kelly 2010). Paying higher amounts for care work means that those who need the care have less money in their already severely limited bank accounts.

Playing one's part in minority politics will exacerbate and multiply problems like the one represented by the direct funding controversy. Christine Kelly argues that models for advocacy must shift and expand: "Advocacy around direct funding must expand in ways that understand personal assistance as 'disabled work,' that is, work that is inherently devalued in our society, just as disabled bodies are" (2010). She further argues:

> One of the ways to transform the cultural meanings of disability is to improve the social status of attendants and the value attributed to their work. There is incredible potential for disabled people to work alongside attendants for the improvement of direct funding programs, but this would require a broadening of identities and mandates endorsed by advocacy groups. (2010)[7]

Kelly here echoes theorist Rosemarie Garland-Thomson's call to consider "disability" a "pervasive cultural category" (2001, 18). Garland-Thomson argues that disability should "be recognized as structuring a wide range of thought, language, and perception that might not be explicitly articulated as 'disability'" (1997). This is a "universalizing rather than minoritizing" move that insists on bridging the binary between disability and ability in a celebration of difference (LaCom 2013). Win contrast, when "disability" is taken up in the context of identity politics that pits one "minority" (marginalized) group against another, opposing lives and labors are devalued and obscured.

Foucault's work provides further theoretical resources to critique minority "disability politics." Adopting roles within the scheme of the minority model involves disability rights advocates directly in the management of their own disability "identity" and the work of policing the border between disability and ability. Seeing "disability" as another minority community pits this group against others in a struggle for rights and access, and further minoritizes and marginalizes persons with disabilities, emphasizing deviance from a norm. In an essay written from a Foucauldian point of view, Helen Liggett notes that "the minority group approach is double-edged because it means enlarging the discursive practices which participate in the constitution of disability . . . in order to participate in their own management disabled people have had to participate as disabled" (Liggett 1988, 271). Shakespeare, meanwhile, argues that "disability politics, by its very nature, often rests on a fairly unreflective acceptance of the disabled/non-disabled distinction. Disabled people are those who identify as such. Disabled leadership is seen as vital" (2006, 78).

RETHINKING DISABILITY: THE CULTURAL MODEL

I turn now to the model that I believe best incorporates insights regarding the play between normality and abnormality and that can avoid problems embedded in the models I have reviewed so far. The *cultural model,* exemplified by the work of Sharon Snyder and David Mitchell, seeks "locations" (contextualized constructions) of disability and deviance. It responds critically to the false choice of *either* the social world *or* the body as an explanatory mechanism. On the one hand, it claims that we can investigate the context and construction of disability without assuming that these contexts and constructions are merely or only tragic or negative—that is, the idea that disability marks "discriminatory encounters" (2006, 10). On the other hand, the cultural model attempts to understand locations of disability as complex interplays between *both* embodiment *and* the social world, and so does not want to exclude individual (negative) experiences of stereotyping and problematic models like the medical model from an understanding of the way that individuals have built their identities (Snyder and Mitchell 2006, 6–7).

This means that the cultural model does not assume that disability is negative, but it can readily incorporate the workings of stigma and prejudice where they occur into an understanding of what disabilities, and disability identities, involve in a variety of contexts. Snyder and Mitchell write: ". . . in keeping with current formulations informed by cultural and identity studies [disability] is largely, but not strictly synonymous with sites of cultural oppression. It does not solely represent the social coordinates, as Liz Crow puts it, of restraints 'that we must escape'" (2006, 6). Snyder and Mitchell go on to clarify that they do not wish to "hide the degree to which social obstacles and biological capacities may impinge upon our lives" (2006, 206).[8]

Their work, instead, recognizes that "environment and bodily variation (especially those traits experienced as socially stigmatized differences) inevitably impinge upon each other" (207).

To reiterate, under the cultural model, defining disability will necessarily involve "a combination of profoundly social and biological forces"—a recipe that neither the medical model nor the social model is able to accommodate (Snyder and Mitchell 2006, 7). Activist and disabled scholar Zola writes: "biology may not determine our destiny; but, as with women, our political, mental and biological differences are certainly part of that destiny" (1993, 170). Recognizing this can lift the veil the social model throws over the body. In this vein, Shakespeare and Erickson write:

> biological and social and cultural processes weave together in complex ways to produce the phenomena which we experience. Just as the best versions of the biological story stress the dynamic processes in nature, the inextricable involvement in the environment with the expression of genes and the crucial role of development, so an adequate social science must acknowledge the bodily and ecological parameters within which humans operate. (2001, 203)

Most importantly, the cultural model is informed by philosophy which can highlight discursive constructions of disability—like Foucault's work—and therefore can interrogate impairment *itself* as socially constructed, as in the case of Shelley Tremain's work (2006). I discuss examples of the social construction of impairment in the next section.

At the outset of this chapter, I mentioned the worry that the reversal strategy of political identity—finding pride in precisely the traits that are stigmatized—was largely unavailable to persons with disabilities. But, the insights of feminist theory, which accord with the cultural model, demonstrate that this kind of reversal is not impossible. Feminist theorist Judy Rohrer, in articulating the entwined interests of feminism and disability theory, points to the strategy of *political ironism*, precisely the type of reversal to which Zola refers.

Rohrer's practice of irony as a political strategy stems from the work of feminist political theorists like Donna Haraway and Kathy Ferguson (2005, 43). Ironism allows one to "live with ambiguity" and, in the words of Ferguson, provides "a way to keep oneself within a situation that resists resolution in order to act politically without pretending that resolution has come" (43). Of disability, Rohrer writes:

> The disabled subject position generates irony through the inescapable friction between living in a disqualified body and *living* at all. Disability is easily understood as a contingent, ambiguous, and multiple category . . . it reminds us of our incompleteness, of the fluidity of our subjectivity, and of the disciplinary practices that shape our bodies and our thinking. (2005, 44)

For Rohrer, irony can "call attention to imposed (mis)representations and new self-definitions while at the same time acknowledging the contingency and fluidity of their identity claims" (44). Rohrer uses "OH" as an example, an acronym which originally refers to "orthopedically handicapped." But, the use of "OH" by persons with disabilities can become a "double gesture" that also signifies "I'm Out-of-Here" (2005, 44). Ironism is a route to reclaim stigmatized identities without negating original meanings; rather, it allows the original meaning to be expressed at the same time as a new meaning, allowing the contrast between the two to yield new space for insight.

Keeping one's eyes open to social construction is an important part of engaging a thickly Foucauldian version of the cultural model. Taking social construction seriously is not the same as engaging a social model of disability. I turn now to describe the social construction of impairment through a series of examples.

Social Constructions of Disability

I consider the meaning of both disability and impairment (as aforementioned, these are often distinguished in an analogy with gender and sex) to be socially conditioned and constructed. This means that strict biological descriptions of disability miss opportunities to critique and analyze the social, political, and other factors that brought them into discourse. I here provide examples of the social constructions of disability, including the influence of genetic determinism.

Susan Wendell points out that there are multiple ways to view the social construction of disability, and the discussion need not be limited to "disability" as a social category while leaving to the side "impairment" as a set of biological categories; in fact, she does not think it is easy to disentangle the two (1996, see esp. Ch. 2). She writes:

> I see disability as socially constructed in ways ranging from social conditions that straightforwardly create illnesses, injuries, and poor physical functioning, to subtle cultural factors that determine standards of normality and exclude those who do not meet them from full participation in their societies. (1996, 58)

For example, political decisions regarding war, the prevention (specifically: the lack of) of violent crime, and differential access to health care can create illness, injury, and therefore have disabling impact (1996, 58–59). These "impairments" are not immune to social construction—indeed, they are "straightforwardly created" by social decisions and are not a mere matter of biology.[9]

Wendell demonstrates that as a professional academic, she stands on shifting sands with regard to her status as a disabled worker at her university;

at the time of her essay, she took one-quarter time disability leave and worked three-quarters time. Increased teaching loads due to changing institutional standards may, she noted, require her to take more disability leave in the future, up to half-time; but nothing about her physical status will have changed (1996, 60). Wendell refers to this constructive phenomenon as "the pace of life,"—that is, changes in standards and expectations which leave persons more or less disabled (59). What most would describe as impairment is here being socially constructed via policy and protocol.

Obesity is another example of the social construction of impairment. Food deserts, poverty, and social inequalities of all types impact rates of "obesity," which many consider a matter of individual responsibility or inherited traits. Definitions of "obesity" and its social meanings are also determined discursively. Ill health is linked to obesity, but many obese persons are in good health. Certain foods are considered "bad" or "good" (fats and dairy are examples) according to evolving standards and changing ideas about what constitutes a healthy diet. Access issues contribute to the idea that persons with disabilities make bad food choices. The need for shopping assistants and prepared foods makes it difficult to obtain and enjoy one's preferred foods, and for those who are able to prepare their own meals, it remains difficult to fulfill the expectations of an increasingly "gourmet" food-centered society and keep up with what some have called "the gentrification of taste" (Gerber 2007). As Elaine Gerber notes, "foods that are easy to prepare or acquire are also often the same ones that deserve criticism for their nutritional shortcomings. Fast foods and pre-prepared foods . . . are the foods that are commonly consumed by disabled people" (Gerber 2007). Meanwhile, food that is considered healthy, green, and organic is precisely the type of food often made inaccessible by contingent social and political factors (poverty, poor urban planning, and "poor architectural planning").

Supposed genetic factors easily frame "fat" as an essential property or a natural kind by connecting being fat with a "fat gene" (Miles 2013). Speaking of sickness and health primarily in terms of biology, or primarily in terms of genetics, obscures and discounts social and political factors structuring ideals of sickness and health; the influence of genetic determinism and other reductions to biology jettisons the philosophically critical chance to analyze and assess these factors and their differential impacts.

Today, the binary between normal and abnormal created by portraits of canonical genotypes and genetic deviance is a key movement of constructions of disability and impairment. In other words, genetic determinism also constructs disability and impairment, especially insofar as it is considered natural, essential, immutable, or adjustable via genetic intervention. Testing procedures which approach testing for mere genetic deviation, that is, the deviation of the genotype of a particular fetus from the genotype of a presumed healthy person, encourage the wrongheaded connection of a type of statistical abnormality to risky embodiment, disability, or illness (see Kelly 2012; Wapner *et al.* 2012). And quality of life predictions based on genetic information taken in utero discount or ignore myriad social, political, and environmental impacts on quality of life and so foreclose potential alternative measures of this concept. All of these processes contribute to the construction of the "impaired fetus" (Tremain 2006). I return to this issue at the end of Chapter 3.

Stigma and Identity

Working within the cultural model, I turn now to stigma. Like Snyder and Mitchell, I seek "locations" of disability. Stigma brings bodily variation to the foreground and so investigating this concept is necessary to arrive at a clearer picture of meanings of disability (in both social and biological senses). It is possible to view disability through a lens of stigma, but also consider physical and mental differences to be the building blocks of disability identities that are not merely negative.

In 1993, disability activist Irving Kenneth Zola produced a brief but canonical essay on the importance of naming and labels, and there adduces a few of the effects that naming can produce for a person with disabilities. Zola claims that "we must go beyond a list of 'do's' and 'don'ts' to an analysis of the functions of [labels]" (1993, 168), and so focuses on function rather than the search for "better" terminology. He argues that labels are both "connotational and associational" (168). First, when one is seen as "sick" or "crazy," a multitude of other traits are brought forward that are frequently associated with illness and madness: "weakness, helplessness, dependency, regressiveness, abnormality of appearance and depreciation of every mode of physical and mental functioning" (168). Second, the label becomes the foundation for explanations of far-flung behavior and signals a set of permanent characteristics:

> Call a person sick or crazy and all their behavior becomes dismissible . . . . Because someone has been labeled ill, all their activity and beliefs—past, present, and future—become related to and explainable in terms of their illness . . . . In the case of a person with a chronic illness and/or a permanent disability, their traits, once perceived to be temporary accompaniments of an illness, become indelible characteristics. (Zola 1993, 168)

Zola also argues that labels have the "potential for spread, pervasiveness, [and] generalization" meaning that the labels come to refer to the person in general and are interpreted in black or white terms. Think here of referencing "the amputee down the hall" or interpreting blindness to mean "totally without vision," something untrue for most blind persons (1993, 169). This links to "spreading effects" more generally. Spread and generalization are central to stigma. Longmore calls this a "spoiling process"; when traits "obscure all other characteristics behind that one and swallow up the social identity of the individual within that restrictive category" (Longmore 1985, 419, quoted in Zola 1993, 169). So, we see here that a trait is emphasized over the whole in situations of labeling. My analysis of transhumanist promotions of new reproductive technologies, which I launch in the next chapter, picks up on this conversation.

Zola argues that grammar produces effects beyond the power of the labels themselves (1993, 170–171). Zola argues that the use of nouns and adjectives ("Blind," "One-Legged") necessarily positions one's trait as primarily important. Nouns "can only perpetuate the equation of the individual equaling the disability. No matter what noun we use, it substitutes one categorical definition for another" (170). Adjectives, meanwhile, "tend to treat the whole person" and are "far from connoting a specific quality of the individual" (170). Prepositions are better (as in "persons with disabilities" and "people of color") primarily *because* they are awkward and create pause; also, the relationships indicated between the terms they combine necessarily separate the terms: prepositions "imply both 'a relationship to' and a 'separation from'" the attribute which is referenced (170). Finally, verbs have both passive and active tenses and so can be limiting; Zola here uses the difference between "using a wheelchair" and "being confined to a wheelchair" to express the distinction (170). The fine distinction between to "have" and "to be" becomes important in these cases, because verbs either "can categorize" or "relate attributes" (170).

Throughout this catalog of grammar, we can see that the political issue is liberating the person described from definition *merely* by way of the disability; this is not a rejection of the trait as negative, but a rejection of definition via the trait, which is unnecessarily limiting. We should use language to express attributes, not to categorize, as Zola suggests. As we shall see in the next chapter, Zola's discussion of labeling and stigma more generally will help us think through how prenatal testing and bioethical discussions of reproductive technology reproduce and deepen stigma.

The concept of stigma can bring into focus spreading effects and the emphasis of traits over persons. Investigating stigma suggests an answer to what kind of community a disability community is. One can consider it a community made up of persons who have experienced the effects of fear, isolation and prejudice on the basis of actual or perceived bodily or mental difference.[10] This is not the end of the possibilities for disability identity, but it is the beginning in today's political context. The medical model has already taught us why the concept of disability is considered exhausted by way of the notion of limitation. But, investigating stigma helps fill out the picture of the disabled subject by suggesting answers to questions that haunt this book—specifically, how does disability become linked with death and fear in bioethics literature?

The mainstay text in disability studies for accounts of stigma is Erving Goffman's sociological study, *Stigma: Notes on the Management of a Spoiled Identity* (1963). According to Snyder and Mitchell, Goffman's "theory of stigma . . . has been influential to cultural model discourses because [it formulates] theories of passing, psychic formation, and materiality as social processes" (2006, 7).[11] Goffman's work takes the notion of stigma from the field of social psychology, and notes that there it is considered "the situation of the individual who is disqualified from full social acceptance" (1963, Preface; cf. 8). Yet, Goffman's work is prescient because of the way in which he receives and adjusts the idea of stigma; he writes that for him, "stigma . . . will be used to refer to an attribute that is deeply discrediting" (1963, 3). So, while acceptance is still at issue, Goffman links the social and the biological in his treatment of stigma. Goffman explicitly addresses spread and generalization by exploring the discrediting effects of certain traits.

Goffman specifies that stigma is produced when there is *lack of fit* between an ideal (in his words: a "virtual" identity) and an actual identity; stigma operates by way of norms (1963, 2–7). Stigma arises "where there is some expectation on all sides that those in a given category should not only support a particular norm but also realize it" (6). The operation of a norm and perceived lack of fit with that norm can produce shame for the individual experiencing stigma (7). More importantly, however, for this discussion, is the social response attracted by the stigmatized lack of fit. Goffman writes: "an individual who might have been received easily in ordinary social intercourse possesses a trait that can obtrude itself upon attention and turn those of us whom he meets away from him, breaking the claim that his other attributes have on us" (5). The presence or absence of a single trait can provide a basis for social rejection that is, at least in part, explicable by way of the "spreading" or "generalization" effect stimulated by that trait.

Goffman argues that others not only "impute" further "imperfections" on the basis of one trait but also tend to assign "some desirable but undesired attributes, often of a supernatural cast, such as 'sixth sense,' or 'understanding'" to those with the "imperfection" (1963, 5). This latter phenomenon should be familiar to anyone who has seen the trope of exceptional wisdom and insight played out on television or the movie screen, an attribute regularly assigned to the ill and dying as well as to the physically or mentally different. Think here of the titular character of Forrest Gump in the 1994 film or John Coffey in *The Green Mile* (1999).

Goffman's articulation of a "trait that can obtrude itself upon attention" is resonant with Adrienne Asch's concept of synecdoche (the identification of a part with a whole). He suggests that in the case of stigma, "imperfections" are assumed on the basis of one trait encountered in another person (1963, 5). Genetic determinism, meanwhile, is also a case of a single trait obtruding upon attention. Furthermore, it is connected to essentializing and naturalizing moves that make particular traits simultaneously highly important and a signal of a "natural kind"—for example, the natural kind of a "disabled" or "defective" person.

Importantly, Goffman helps the able-bodied see themselves as "temporarily able-bodied" (TAB) and rejects false binaries between abled and disabled precisely by way of his analysis of stigma. He notes that although one may not already be discredited, one can always be interpreted as *discreditable*:

> The most fortunate of normals is likely to have [their] half-hidden failing, and for every little failing there is a social occasion when it will loom large, creating a shameful gap between virtual and actual social identity. Therefore the occasionally precarious and the constantly precarious form a single continuum, their situation in life analyzable by the same framework. (1963, 127)

We can read the echoes of Goffman in the work of Garland-Thomson and her discussion of the normate, the empty cultural ideal that no one person can fulfill (1996, 9).

Drawing on Goffman's work, Lerita Coleman Brown argues that "stigma is a response to the dilemma of difference" (2010, 179). She writes: "What is most poignant about Goffman's description of stigma is that it suggests that *all human differences* are potentially stigmatizable" (179, emphasis mine). This is why disability is a fundamentally unstable category. So, for Coleman Brown (as well as for Goffman), "stigmas reflect the value judgments of a dominant group" (180). With a turn, again, to social psychology, Coleman Brown categorizes stigma as a mode of "cognitive processing" which helps us categorize and respond to difference (183). But, she is especially intent to argue that the *fear* so often involved in stigma is a complex affective response specifically expressive of learned behaviors: "interest and curiosity about stigma or human differences may be natural for children, but they must *learn* fear and avoidance as well as which categories or attributes to dislike, fear, or stigmatize . . . certain negative emotions become attached to social categories" (183). *Stigma thinking* for Coleman Brown is thus deeply connected to schemas and stereotyping.

For Coleman Brown, stigma is a "special and insidious kind of social categorization" which is a "process of generalizing from a single experience" (2010, 184). Like Goffman, she argues that stigma is "the attribute that colors the perception of the entire person" and "other aspects of the person are ignored" (184). Overall, for Coleman Brown, stigma "maintains" the status quo of social relations and brings stigmatized and unstigmatized persons "together in a perpetual inferior/superior relationship" (184, 185, and 189). This binary is maintained despite Goffman's insight that stigmatization exists on a continuum to which no one is immune (cf. Coleman Brown 2010, 187). Examining stigma reveals the openness all have to stigmatization, given the fact of human difference. But, stigma can only maintain itself through the encouragement of social exclusions and support of the status quo.

It is clear that to be stigmatized is undesirable. But, Coleman Brown helps us glean slightly more from the concept of stigma when she suggests that stigma causes fear because it is, at root, "uncontrollable"—"human differences serves as the basis for stigmas" and so one can be stigmatized at any time (2010, 187). In that sense, Coleman Brown argues, the structure of stigma imitates the structure of death:

> The unpredictability of stigma is similar to the unpredictability of death . . . the development of a stigmatized condition in a loved one or in oneself represents a major breach of trust—a destruction of the belief that life is predictable. In a sense, stigma represents a kind of death—a social death . . . nonstigmatized people, through avoidance and social rejection, often treat stigmatized people as if they were invisible, nonexistent, or dead. (188)

The linkage between stigma and death does not stop there, especially when stigmatized traits are precisely traits that remind us of human vulnerability or mortality. As Coleman Brown argues, "many stigmas, in particular childhood cancer, remove the visual disguises of mortality. Such stigmas can act as a symbolic reminder of everyone's inevitable death" (2010, 188). At this point it should be clear that to those who would seek immortality, like transhumanists, stigmatized persons could represent a particularly painful reminder—the existence of these individuals is painted as inevitably risky.

Exclusions and stigma which accompany bodily difference are very strict (cf. Goffman 1963, 127–128). Ectrodactyly and syndactyly, which result in missing fingers and toes and the "partial fusion of the bones of the fingers and toes," may seem relatively insignificant over the course of a life (Parens and Asch 2000, 8). But, when Bree Walker Lampley, a news personality who had both these traits, called ectrodactyly "minor" and stated her intention to continue a pregnancy although she knew the resulting child would have that particular trait, the media was scandalized and she was widely criticized as "irresponsible" (9). This is intelligible only within biopolitical and eugenic logic. Another testament to the stringency of stigma is the fact that, as Goffman argues, a stigma which has been "repaired" or "corrected" is still a limiting stigma. She writes: "where such repair is possible, what often results is not the acquisition of fully normal status, but a transformation of self from someone with a particular blemish into someone with a record of having corrected a particular blemish" (1963, 9). The faintest whiff of deviance from the norm is enough for the pernicious effects of stigma to operate; this speaks to the strength of operative norms and biopolitical logic. Stigma can attach to any perceived difference, yet difference (as opposed to identity) is everywhere.

CONCLUSION

While issues of disability identity and disability models are of course not resolved by way of my analysis and discussion here, I would note that it is fully consistent with Rohrer's political ironism and with Foucault's legacy to accept the ambiguity surrounding disability. Doing so is also a testament to the important linkages between feminism and disability theory, both of which are politically responsive. Both also seek ultimately to critique the status quo; along those lines, to analyze stigma as part of disability identities is not to resign oneself to the idea that disability is merely negative. In the next chapter, I go on to deploy the cultural model in a historical investigation of the many meanings of disability as determined by a history of enhancement thinking. Foucault's genealogical model, which uncovers the play between norms and deviance and treats the body as the locus of history, provides me with the framework I need. Today's genetic definitions of normality and abnormality, health and deviance, are an important front line of stigmatizing responses to what Coleman Brown calls the "dilemma of difference" (2010, 179). In what follows, I trace these cleavages in their place, as descendants in a genealogy of enhancement thinking. As I continue to argue in the remainder of this book, reductions to the biological, including genetic reductions, miss the many meanings of disability and undercut the well-being of disabled persons by stigmatizing, isolating, and excluding them—even to the point of death.

NOTES

1. I analyze this matter in a discussion of vile sovereignty and transhumanism in Hall 2013.

2. For complete analysis of the Supreme Court Case in which a deaf public elementary student was denied an interpreter, see Anita Silvers' discussion of *Board of Education of the Hendrick Hudson Central School District* v *Rowley* (2009, 180–181).

3. Sandra Bartky also describes this kind of cultural isolation for women, given that they live with men and take on patriarchal culture as their own (2005).

4. I cannot, of course, be exhaustive here in my consideration of models of disability; an example of a model I do not consider is the "consumer" model, which would position persons with disabilities as an untapped market (cf. Riley 2005).

5. I engage the use of disability in horror, and the possibilities for liberating visions of disability in horror, in Hall 2016.

6. Scott-Hill is also published under the name "Mairian Corker."

7. This connects with Eva Kittay's call for "doulia": "Just as we have required care to survive and thrive, so we need to provide conditions that allow others—including those who do the work of caring—to receive the care they need to survive and thrive" (1999, 68, cf. 107). Care work is devalued by its proximity to the cared-for, and both are locked together until a critique of this devaluation can pull them apart.

8. In other words, they speak to the following concern articulated by Susan Wendell: "I do not think that my body *is* a cultural representation, although I recognize that my experience of it is both highly interpreted and very influenced by cultural (including medical) interpretations" (1996, 62).

9. Wendell also describes the more familiar social construction of disability that the social model can easily recognize: "poor architectural planning creates physical obstacles for people who use wheelchairs, but also for people who can walk but cannot walk far or cannot climb stairs, for people who cannot open doors, or for people who can do all these things but only at the cost of pain or an expenditure of energy they can ill afford" (1996, 60–61).

10. The text of the Americans with Disabilities Act has the issue of perception built in to its definition of disability, claiming disability status for persons who are perceived to have a disability trait. "The term 'disability' means with respect to an individual (a) a physical or mental impairment that substantially limits one or more of the major life activities of such an individual; (b) a record of such an impairment; (c) being *regarded* as having such an impairment" (ADA quoted in Riley 2005, 7; emphasis mine).

11. Snyder and Mitchell give similar priority to Judith Butler's work on "sex/gender binaries" (2006, 7). In this chapter, I speak briefly to the problems tied to the attempted analogy by the DRM and other activist groups between sex/gender and impairment/disability, but further discussion is outside the scope of this project.

Chapter 3

Rethinking Enhancement

A Genealogical Approach

In this chapter, I argue that, in a continuation of enhancement strategies repeated throughout the twentieth century, transhumanism operates by performing biological reductions and engaging in biopolitical logic. That is, transhumanism reduces questions of social change to a discussion of altering the body and rejecting deviant bodies. Transhumanists, like many enhancement enthusiasts across the last century, do not question the assumption that social problems root from natural circumstances, when in fact they can be traced to social and political decision-making. It is important to historicize social contexts, disability, and calls for enhancement, and to fight this naturalization.[1] I do so in this chapter by calling explicitly on Foucault's method of genealogy.

Foucault's understanding of genealogy is laid out in "Nietzsche, Genealogy, and History" (1977). There, he describes the genealogical method, which he draws from Nietzsche: "Genealogy does not oppose itself to history as the lofty and profound gaze of the philosopher might compare to the mole-like perspective of the scholar; on the contrary, it rejects the metahistorical deployment of ideal significations and indefinite teleologies. It opposed itself to the search for 'origins'" (77). Indeed, Foucault is reading Nietzsche here as a critic of the *ursprung* or origin, because it seeks "the exact essence of things" and is too faithful to a mistaken metaphysics (78). Genealogy is entangled, messy, and involves tracing "jolts and surprises," rather than teleological unfolding (80). This type of history-telling "operates on a field of entangled and confused parchments, on documents that have been scratched over and recopied many times" (76). When Nietzsche examines "the history of reason, he learns that it was born in an altogether 'reasonable' fashion—from chance" (78); "historical beginnings are lowly . . . derisive and ironic, capable of undoing every infatuation" (79).

Within the genealogical method, history is made concrete; and the body is revealed as a locus for history:

> The body is the inscribed surface of events (traced by language and dissolved by ideas), the locus of a dissociated self (adopting the illusion of a substantial unity), and a volume in perpetual disintegration. Genealogy, as an analysis of descent, is thus situated within the articulation of the body and history. Its task is to expose a body totally imprinted by history and the process of history's destruction of the body. (1977, 83)

Telling genealogical history, then, is not a metaphysical matter of teleology, but rather records the particular traces of events on the body and chasing of the body as a "perpetually disintegrating" volume.

In this chapter, I investigate the historical setting and influencing factors of today's bioethical debate over human enhancement technologies by way of a cultural and historical genealogy of enhancement strategies in the twentieth century. I consider rhetoric in three key historical moments: physical culture at the turn of the century, the birth of the field of endocrinology in the 1910s and 1920s, and post–Second World War rehabilitations of eugenic thinking in the 1950s. I find recurring, persistent biological reductions and discover that the structure of ableism—discrimination against persons with stigmatized traits—shifts and changes along with conceptions of health. Social and cultural prejudices become strategies for distinguishing between the sick and the healthy, the good and the bad body, and the good and the bad mind. Enhancement rhetoric feeds from these distinctions and I expose the surrounding rhetoric as a marginalizing discourse. I end the chapter by outlining genetic determinism, which is endemic to contemporary transhumanist thinking and connected in character to the biological reductions performed repeatedly in the twentieth century.

I see my work in this chapter as similar in spirit to that of Licia Carlson in *The Faces of Intellectual Disability* (2009), in which she provides a genealogical history (or what she calls a historical ontology) inspired by Foucault, of the evolution and development of the concept of "mental retardation." She explores the ways intellectual disability is set up against portraits of "normal" cognition (xv, 1–2, 14). Her work acts against the naturalization of mental retardation as a human kind.

THE LIFE EXTENSION INSTITUTE

In 1913, a group of American philanthropic celebrities, politicians, and scientists founded the Life Extension Institute, which—as its name suggests—aimed to prolong human life. President William H. Taft, who had just completed his term in office, was Chairman of the Board of Directors and Dr. William J. Mayo, who six years later helped found the Mayo Clinic, was a member of the Institute's Hygiene Board. Scientists Irving Fisher and Eugene Fisk co-authored the Institute's major tract, entitled *How to Live: Rules for Healthful Living Based on Modern Science* (1916). As the group's most prominent member, President Taft wrote the Foreword for *How to Live* and makes the biopolitical claim that health is the primary end of politics. He writes, "the care of individual and family health is the first and most patriotic duty of a citizen" (viii). *How to Live* discusses diet, exercise, deep breathing, and hygiene. It recommends "thorough mastication" (Chapter 2, Section 4) and good posture (Chapter 3, "Poisons," Sec 2). But, Fisher and Fisk do not ultimately conclude that physical health and morality can be left up to individual behavior; instead, they considered health and morality heritable and therefore argued that a "thoroughgoing eugenic program" was needed for "society as a whole" (167). The Life Extension Institute sets the scene for discourse around enhancement strategies and population health in the twentieth century.

Less benign than chewing and posture, then, were the tract's directives regarding marriage and reproduction, as in a section entitled "Comparison of Degenerative Tendencies Among Nations" (Fisher and Fisk 1916, 286–292), a concluding section on eugenics which recommended both forced sterilization (323, cf. 167), and the works of eugenics figurehead Sir Francis Galton (296). In 1869, Galton set in motion an international discussion of parental duties with regard to heritable traits (Buchanan *et al.* 2000, 30–31; Snyder and Mitchell 2006, 25). Echoing him, Fisher and Fisk see morality and immorality as determined by "family lines"—and the swath of traits they identify among this set is breathtaking:

> Moral Traits.—Among the moral traits known to possess inheritable elements are generosity, piousness, independence, industry, will-power, faithfulness, fairness, sociability, reliability, self-reliance, tendency to work hard, perseverance, carefulness, impulsiveness, temperance, high-spiritedness, joviality, benignity, quietness, cheerfulness, hospitality, sympathy, humorousness, love of fun, neighborliness, love of frontier life, love of travel and of adventure. The same may be said of immoral traits, such as criminality, pauperism, delinquency, irascibility, lying, truancy, superstition, clannishness, secretiveness, despondency, slyness, exclusiveness, vanity, cunning, cruelty, quickness to anger, revengefulness, etc. (1916, 298)

Notice, just as in the case of today's enhancement advocacy, happiness ("high-spiritedness"; recall the "zest" to which Nick Bostrom refers) and use-value ("industry") were taken as a biological matter which could be increased by (then proto-) genetic choice-making. The contemporary reader will notice especially items like "love of frontier life, love of travel and of adventure" as constructed by social expectations at the time of writing—an enduring social legacy of America's manifest destiny doctrine and American exceptionalism. But, for Fisher and Fisk, this list of traits is based on a highly objective standard:

> The question of what traits are desirable and what traits are undesirable might seem, on first thought, rather a difficult matter to determine. Few of us would like to have our neighbor's taste in the matter constituted as a standard of judgment upon our own traits. There is one standard of judgment, however, that is so broad and impersonal . . . that it can justly serve as a line of division between the desirability and undesirability . . . This is the measurement by the standard of social worth and service commonly designated as "fitness." (1916, 300–301)

Fisher and Fisk's discussion of fitness divides populations into two groups; the fit are those "who are a service to society, or at least not a burden" while the unfit are "a burden: economically and socially" (1916, 301). Fisher and Fisk mark traits as desirable *after* the individual who holds them is identified as "not a burden for others" (which is why they can juxtapose carefulness and impulsiveness), but they have stereotypes of social undesirability ready to hand: "the feeble-minded, paupers, criminals, insane, weak and sick" (301).

How to Live becomes a question of living *without* the feeble minded, and the biopolitical logic is obvious. The frontispiece of *How to Live* reads: "Prevent Life-Waste—Upbuild National Vitality." At the turn of the century, the health of a population is considered dependent upon eliminating the influence of "sick" members (Life-Waste). In this way, health and morality were linked to regulating reproduction and segregation on the level of the population and to the discipline of the body through hygiene and diet on the level of the individual. Marriage was brought under scrutiny as a result. The implication was that "bad" marriages involving the unfit will result in a bad society because they would produce defective offspring. These themes were supported in eugenics propaganda films like *Are You Fit to Marry?* (1927, first released as *The Black Stork* in 1917). Besides outright sterilization, Fisher and Fisk argue for the segregation of persons considered defective and—in addition to "wise marriage laws"—the "development of an enlightened sentiment against improper marriages" (1916, 167).

In continuation with the Institute, life extension remains a primary goal of enhancement enthusiasts today (Bostrom 2005a; 2008, 113–116; Harris 2004, Heard 1997, Shostak 2002). Morality is still considered heritable and manipulable through science and technology. In fact, significant recent writing in bioethics includes calls to improve human beings morally and socially through scientific and technological means (Buchanan 2011a, 2011b, Liao *et al.* 2012, Persson and Savulescu 2011, 2012). For example, transhumanist and bioethicist Julian Savulescu argues that bad tempers should be curbed through genetic selection (2001b). Bioethicist Allen Buchanan argues for enhancement of the capacity for impulse control and sympathy, among other valued social traits, and Bostrom argues that it is important to enhance human capability with regard to "appropriate affect," among other issues connected to sensibility (Buchanan 2011 and Bostrom 2008, 108 and 2009).

It is possible to analyze these current issues through a history of eugenic thought culminating with the German Nazi regime and Nazi medicine during WWII. Many invaluable scholarly works outline the history of attempts to remake the human body and improve it with direct reference to the eugenic ideology which surfaced in the German Nazi regime—but which, of course, is rooted in much earlier history (e.g. Kevles 1985; Paul 1995; Proctor 1988). Scholars have shown that continuous and recent attitudes toward the centrality of genetics or the rejection of persons with "marked bodies" are in line with or provided a basis for Nazi ideology (Bauman 1989, Kerr and Shakespeare 2002; Kittay 2010a; Kröner 1999; Snyder and Mitchell 2006, esp. Chapter 2; cf. Mitchell and Snyder 2000, ix). Indeed, Foucault sees in the Nazi regime the perfection of the state-sponsored racism at the root of biopower (2003b, 259).

But, instead of pursuing a direct critique of eugenics, done excellently in the books cited above and elsewhere, I seek to develop the conversation by tracing rhetoric surrounding enhancement. I follow the example of disability theorists Sharon Snyder and David Mitchell who argue that Nazi ideology is *continuous* with modernism rather than an exception and that we all lose when we assume that excessive hardship and deviance are embedded in embodiment itself (2006, 5). Zygmunt Bauman, likewise, sees Nazi eugenics as a continuation rather than an aberration of modernist projects (1989). An important part of these modernist projects, which are still manifest today in transhumanism, is the "[promise] to rid the land of all defectives" (Snyder and Mitchell 2006, 79). As Snyder and Mitchell put it, this promise is tied up in a "uniquely modern utopian fantasy of a future world uncontaminated by defective bodies" (129). This is the precisely the transhumanist fantasy which guides my discussion in this book, but I want to focus on the political technologies of the present that attempt to bring it about.

In what follows, then, I describe and explore neglected aspects of eugenic history that prefigure and situate current enhancement promotion. In the three moments I consider, I highlight the following biopolitical elements: 1) lasting commitments to a particular kind of discipline and transcendence of the body, 2) the equation of physical and mental health, both of individuals and populations, with morality, happiness and sociability, and 3) continuous reference to and reconstruction of what counts as a deviant body. The alternative eugenic history I draw should act as layering scenes, which slowly unravel issues attending biological reductions of all kinds. Though the content and meanings of biological reductions shift and build over time, I see the genetic reduction committed by transhumanists today as deeply connected to history. Ultimately, the structure of genetic determinism underlying transhumanist rhetoric is revealed in the historical moments I explore. To begin, I visit "physical culture" to reveal what, at that time, fell under the as yet untarnished banner of eugenics.

PHYSICAL CULTURE, DISCIPLINE, AND HEALTHY CHOICES

Against the backdrop of the focus on heritability and social and personal hygiene exemplified by the aims and status of the Life Extension Institute, physical culture flourished at the turn of the century in the United States and in Europe. The physical culture movement, inherited from the Victorians, emphasized exercise, body-building, and hygiene. A popular magazine entitled *Physical Culture*, founded in 1899, enjoyed a print run lasting through the 1940s (Bennett 2012). Exploring the pages of this popular magazine illuminates the rhetorical stakes of physical culture. *Physical Culture* magazine was most likely inspired by a similar earlier publication in Britain produced by Eugen Sandow, a Prussian bodybuilder present at the World's Columbia Exposition in Chicago in 1893. President Theodore Roosevelt also influenced the physical culture movement of which Sandow was a symbol through advocacy of the "strenuous life" and its power over his own childhood sickness (Fair 2012).

The magazine, which (in line with the Life Extension Institute's recommendations) promoted diet, exercise, sunlight, and cleanliness as a formula for a happy life, declared: "every influence which interferes with the attainment of superb, buoyant health should be recognized as menace" (1934, 63). In other words, one must aggressively self-regulate in order to protect one's health from continuous threat. But, physical culture was not merely about body-building and the wonders of strenuous exercise for overcoming disease.

Albert Wiggam, a frequent contributor to *Physical Culture* magazine, declared a new standard for choosing a marriage partner, and partner reproducer, derived from the knowledge of biologists. In an article entitled "Wanted: A Eugenics Conscience," he writes that parents should "be carrying healthy, happy and congenial germ-cells from their ancestors and, thus, be capable of transmitting healthy, happy and congenial bodies and minds to their children" (Wiggam 1934, 16). The wrong partner can be a "menace" to the "attainment of superb, buoyant health" and so too can one's parents; one might lose the chance for happiness if the wrong match (genetic choice) is made. Meanwhile a physically healthy parent could set their children up for life. So writes *Physical Culture* reader Mrs. Earl Wood, from Detroit, Michigan in 1934: "When I was born into this world, my mother had bestowed upon me one of the greatest gifts of life—perfect health" (6). Mrs. Wood must mean what Doctor X, later in the same issue, calls "an *intelligence of the physique*" which he worries has gone by the wayside but would have "won laurels and plaudits" in a "simpler, more heroic society" such as ancient Greece (15).

This constitutes a call to Americans to strengthen their culture—lurking in the background is a cult of national vitality. But, notice that this "intelligence of the physique" is not merely a set of physical attributes, but also attributes of mind, mood and attitude: that is, "healthy, happy and congenial bodies and minds," according to Wiggam. So we see, again, that happiness, health, and therefore social congeniality is treated as heritable and therefore manipulable through proto-genetic choice-making—but also depends later upon choosing physical exercise, diets, and vitamins. Physical culture explicitly linked physical health and discipline with choice-making, responsibility, and moral goodness, and delineated and denigrated threatening, dangerous outsiders which must be dealt with: those characterized as the sick and the weak.

In the 1934 issue of *Physical Culture*, a stricken father reported the events of his son's birth. According to the doctor, something was wrong: "'There's a defect here!' The doctor cried sharply to the midwife. 'Defective heart action!'" (12). The father wrote about his own heart problems and felt anxiety with regard to passing along the condition: "[The doctor's words were] like a dagger of remorse to me for I thought I had done the unpardonable—transmitted my own bad heart to my son" (12). The mention of unpardonable action is no accident—according to the rhetoric of physical culture, bad health was truly a crime. A motto printed on the front cover of the June 1947 issue of *Physical Culture* and repeated in other issues clarifies the point: "Sickness is a sin: Don't be a sinner" and "Weakness is a crime: Don't be a criminal." The sick and the weak, then, constituted a population of undesirables who were both sinful and criminal, threatening the health of all with their bad choices. Between the medical professional and the father in this (likely fictional) story is the hinge between disciplinary and regulatory mechanisms that make up the operation of biopower.

Bernarr Macfadden, founder of the magazine, wrote the above magazine mottos and authored dozens of books about physical culture. Macfadden figured the relationship between abnormality and criminality as running both ways (Adams 2009; Ernst 1991). He claimed that criminals "are all abnormal—there are but few exceptions" (Macfadden 1934, 4). This violent pairing is not unfamiliar to anyone versed in racist and ableist eugenic ideology, and recalls Foucault's discussion of criminal prehistories of abnormality in *Abnormal* (2003a, 21–23). Macfadden goes on: "If we owned a cat or a dog, or any domestic animal, that was deformed and misshapen as is the average 'human,' it would not be considered worth keeping and death would end its earthly pilgrimage" (1934, 4). Macfadden declares that life is not worth living for some and claims for this judgment call a kind of biological objectivity. He asks and answers the biopolitical question: Who should live?

In another article in *Physical Culture*, Wiggam again calls for a "eugenics conscience," this time a bit more directly. Here, he asks, in line with Macfadden: "Shall We Breed or Sterilize Defectives?" (1934, 16). Who should live? Wiggam calls upon the authority of eugenicist Charles Davenport of the Carnegie Institution in order to argue that "migrating families" of "gypsies" ought to be sterilized so that valuable social resources could be saved—eliminating this threat means enhancement for the whole population (16–17). He is aghast that some object to sterilization for those populations and individuals he considers undesirable and writes:

> If such persons [who would object to sterilization] would turn and consider the money expended on these worthless breeds, which ought to be used and could be used to educate and furnish jobs for their own children it would seem that this alone would answer all their objections. If they further would consider the moral corruption in addition to the havoc wrought by the spread of disease that I have myself witnessed many times in a community brought about by the sex-looseness of some good-looking feebleminded or moron girl, again it would seem this would answer their objections. (17)[2]

In this excerpt, cost—benefit analysis are plainly layered upon pronouncements regarding the immorality or a-morality of deviant bodies and populations. The space of the clinic in which these sterilizations occurred becomes the space in which utopian fantasies were enacted with disciplinary interventions justified by reference to the safety of the population. Today, similarly, the feasibility and desirability of incurring medical costs of caring for persons with disabilities is laid open for debate; this is often placed in a context of health-care rationing. Julian Savulescu considers this question with regard to cardiac care and persons with Down syndrome, concluding that triage is necessary because resources are limited and therefore equality of access is not as attractive as it might seem (2001c). Medical resources are often redirected away from disabled persons, who have a much greater level of difficulty accessing medical resources (e.g. Chandler *et al.* 2006). The refusal of transplants for persons with disabilities is a regular problem (Cohen 2013).

Although Wiggam brings himself to note that not all the "feeble-minded and moron people" he has in mind are "necessarily bad," he quickly establishes that, if nothing else, "they are *all irresponsible people*."[3] The linkage of personal irresponsibility—that is, *bad choice-making*—with the sick and the weak, along with the rehabilitation on the level of the population of an underlying "defective" genotype which must be destroyed, is repeated earnestly in founding theological-bioethical texts of the 1970s (Passmore 1970, Ramsey 1970).

Those who used prosthetic devices or were in other ways dependent were also figured as irresponsible and lazy. One advertisement in *Physical Culture* magazine admonished readers that "Eye-glasses Never Mar the Faces of Beauty Contest Winners" and reminded them, in skewed fonts, that "Glasses are only Eye-Crutches—anyway." A coupon is offered so that (especially women, who are pictured) can "throw the glasses away." The secret was training exercises for the eyes, which should be taken up in order to avoid dependence on a "crutch" (1934, 8).

While much was blamed on heritability in *Physical Culture* magazine, which I am taking as expressive of the physical culture movement's mores, exercise and vitamins were simultaneously posed as restorative health measures that should be pursued by choice-makers under banner of independence. For example, the father worried over transmitting a "bad heart" to his newborn child watched as the doctor sprang into action; he "began swinging the baby up and down like a calisthenics drill," a procedure which, combined with "smack[ing] him brutally" and dips in hot and cold water eventually produced a "heart-gladdening little wail!" (1934, 13). Indeed, (uncomfortable) exercises were meant to be extended to infants, according to the tracts of physical culture (Macfadden published, with wife Marguerite, *Physical culture for babies*, 1904) and were considered extremely important at such a formative time. This particular father spent the infant's childhood engaged in a struggle between the food of Old Europe introduced by the child's mother, who was not American and urged travel abroad, and the vitamins the father introduced. Notice the rhetorical linkages here between: women and unhealthy heredity, America and physical vitality, and the father with rational and healthy choice-making. The child's health problems, however, were eventually remedied by a return to U.S. soil from abroad and a practice of pressing his legs together and holding him upside down "by his heels" (13, 82). Rough calisthenics were enough to soothe the inherited "defective heart" and, one presumes, make a true American of the child.

In another example of "choosing health," vitamins were suggested as an ameliorative tool for deafness in the April 1940 issue of *Physical Culture*. Dr. Emanuel Josephson argues in "New Hope for the Deaf" that "one of the best methods of increasing the body's resistance to ear infections and of restoring hearing to a high and efficient level is by means of a vitamin-rich diet" (10). And, in a move familiar from today's "supercrip" stories of inspirational physical achievement (Clare 1999, 2–9, cf. Diane DeVries's childhood as explored in Frank 2000), choosing exercise is recommended for infantile paralysis by the notable example of a beautiful young girl: "stricken with infantile paralysis at the age of eight, Nancy Merki is today the proud holder of three national swimming records, and one world's championship. Here is the inspiring story of a courageous youngster who literally swam her way from invalidism to buoyant health and world fame" (14). Physical discipline, then, involves transcendence—the transcendence and overcoming of the pains of embodiment. To have a disability meant that one was not taking one's vitamins or daily swim—one had refused to discipline one's body, and was, ultimately, threatening the population.

Throughout the turn of the century and the rise of physical culture, alongside a growing knowledge of genetics and attention paid to heredity, choosing vitamins and exercise played a prominent role in the public imagination with regard to health from the turn of the twentieth century. Sickness and weakness, as sin and as crime, could be blamed on an "irresponsible" parent who passes on inferior (read: dis-abled, raced, classed, sexed) traits, *and* someone who has not demonstrated the get-up-and-go necessary to overcome physical or mental difference or who refuses to avail themselves of the maximizing benefits of vitamins and sunlight. A variety of traits, both individual and social, were reduced to facts about the body. One could choose the correct marriage partner, thereby ensuring future happiness, and choose to enhance one's body through vitamins and exercise, thereby ensuring ability against the threat of disability and gaining access to a future of "buoyant health and world fame." The *choice-maker* is thus the figure of health, strength, and morality, and we continue to attempt to arrange ourselves as such.

Key features of physical culture persist in today's enhancement debate, especially among transhumanists and other advocates of radical enhancement. The valorization of certain bodies and circumstances is based in and justifies the rejection of other bodies; after all, one must protect one's health against the menace others pose, especially if that menace is an entire community who refuses to make rational choices (e.g. Wiggam's reaction to the Roma, who were expected to live in permanent exile and stop reproducing). Shared society in one's community and in one's home today becomes a shared gene pool, and we are warned that the danger is more insidious than ever—we cannot tolerate deviance, or we might go extinct (Savulescu 2009, Persson and Savulescu 2013). Parents must be responsible choosers and so must their children.

THE BIRTH OF ENDOCRINOLOGY

Continuing my exploration of the last century of enhancement thinking, I turn now to a second moment which yields another complex strategy of enhancement and new separations of the deviant from the healthy. The birth and acceptance of the field of endocrinology ushered in a fresh conception of the human being as *hormonal*, a move which adds to and deepens the convictions of the physical culture movement and its fetishism of appropriate marriages, diet, and exercise. Here, we still have a reduction to the biological, but there is a renewed sense of the biological. Discourses of diagnosis and calls to action shape-shift and reorganize.

Endocrinology gained traction in the 1910s and 20s (Rothman and Rothman 2003, 13). Because of the importance of new ventures in endocrinology within the venture-capitalist context of medicine, hormones and endocrinology were ready to play a public role now filled by gene-editing procedures (13). Endocrinology promised to wage war against aging and infertility. In popular discourse, hormones replaced the vitamins and sunlight of the physical culture days while maintaining focus on heredity that would eventually give over to the discussion of genes in today's discourse and medical climate. The discovery and exploration of the activity of hormones emphasized biological influence upon human lives above all. Reinforcing and reconstructing the category of the criminally weak and sinfully malnourished of physical culture, "freaks" became "patients with glandular irregularities who required medical care" (18).

This discourse conjures up images of the suppression and transcendence of the influence of freakish hormonal outsiders, who, if they were not eliminated or somehow enhanced, threaten the progress of all. Again, enhancement for all requires the regulation of particular individuals. Hormone deficiency became the scapegoat for all manner of ills—including, most importantly, perceived issues in growth, puberty, fertility, and aging. In the case of growth and puberty, speed was desired; in the case of fertility, enhancement; and in the case of aging, deceleration. The hormonal conversation brought into play at the very least a desire to move beyond the existence of short "freaks" (today's enhancement conversation is still rife with masculinist concern regarding achieving height) and some began to envision a renewed world populated by giants. Herbert George Wells writes of this vision in 1926:

> A time will come when littleness will have passed altogether out of the world of man. When giants shall go freely about this earth—their earth—doing continually greater and more splendid things. But, that—is to come. We are not even the first generation of that—we are the first experiment. (21)

Wells' conceptual structure echoes the reaction of Wiggam to "gypsies"—defectives, outside the freshened and bolstered notion of the normal body, are unwelcome in a world where the norm can flourish. The defective is seen to clamp down upon and preclude the potential of the norm. This is deviance reconfigured, a persistent and continuously updated notion of who fails to earn a place in the world and who should be pushed out of it. Again, we have a menace, and again, answers to the question of who should live. As Foucault puts it, biopolitics teaches that "the very fact that you let more die will allow you to live more" (2003b, 255).

Endocrinology drove an effort to isolate masculine and feminine "principles" and use these essences to stave off the unwanted effects of aging and remedy infertility for the upper classes. This drive was supported by profit-seeking pharmaceutical companies (Rothman and Rothman 2003). Companies like Eli Lilly, working closely in fateful collaboration with university researchers from institutions like the University of Toronto and Johns Hopkins (and slaughterhouses, which provided animal corpses for use in the research), hawked largely untried and unproven remedies among physicians (13, 32–34, 47). This was the venture capitalism of endocrinology. Physicians reported high levels of confidence in the pharmaceutical employees who visited them with new products, and these "detail men" cynically produced guidance pamphlets with instructions on socializing with medical professionals for profit (47).

New institutional collaborations had major effects upon the diagnosis, treatment, and experience of patients. Diagnoses related to hormonal "deficiencies" abounded. For example, "shortness of stature" became a diagnosis and "the very short child" was suddenly seen by the medical establishment as "a sick child" (Rothman and Rothman 2003, 173–174). Medical historians Rothman and Rothman relate this to contemporary questions in bioethics regarding the line between cure and enhancement; they note that new technologies define new disease states in those once considered normal (174). Endocrinology as a discourse picked up on latent notions of fitness and heredity. In the past century of enhancement thinking, faults, diagnoses, and fixes are written across the body as disciplinary and regulatory power techniques define norms.

Physicians prescribed what are now known as testosterone and estrogen to patients, using negative techniques to determine the usefulness or necessity of the prescriptions. If the patient—having received these remedies—experienced improvement vis-à-vis their complaints, the patient had a deficiency of testosterone or estrogen (Rothman and Rothman 2003, 31). These patient-reported improvements justified the treatment plan. The same strategy of diagnosis-by-trial was later used in the case of the development of human growth hormone (HGH) (180–181). Faced with the advertisement rhetoric of potential deficiency and the promise of a better life, patients were desperate for access to the drugs. This rhetoric acts in parallel to the utopia of the transhumanist—who can say no to increased happiness, or to the "best life" for one's child? Hormonal influence received a cathexis of hope with regard to staving off age and maintaining health. Here we see that definitions of deviance and health are continually updated, shifting shape and deepening—that is, moving deeper within the body—over time.

POSTWAR REHABILITATION OF EUGENIC IDEALS

I turn now to the post–Second World War attempt to rehabilitate eugenic ideas and the construction of a specifically genetic version of normality and abnormality. This discourse takes for granted that the body is an appropriate location for intervention in order to alleviate some social ills—it performs yet another version of a biological reduction and moves even deeper within the body. Additionally, as we shall see, it is a direct ancestor (although not a pure origin point) of today's transhumanist thinking and indulges in the genetic visions that reverberate today.

The rejection of the exposed genocidal policies and eugenic practices of the Third Reich in the mid-twentieth century changed the topography of academia in the United States (Buchanan *et al.* 2000, 37–40). As is now well known, prior to WWII, North American and European eugenicists cited one another as academic and legislative resources (Snyder and Mitchell 2006; Buchanan *et al.* 2000, 38). After the war, U.S. scientists and social theorists distanced themselves from the discredited eugenic label. This post war rejection transformed academic journals and societies previously explicitly dedicated to aspects of eugenics (Buchanan *et al.* 2000, 39).

But, philosophical and social-scientific moves were made to rehabilitate eugenics from its bad reputation. Julian Huxley, for example, denied that eugenics must fall to Nazi ills.[4] In essays collected under the title *Man in the Modern World*, Huxley—trained as a biologist—expressed a desire to affect public policy to improve modern life (1948). In fact, it was Huxley who first coined the word "transhumanism" prior to WWII (in 1927) and was its advocate into the 1950s. He believed transcendence of typical human bounds was important—and such transcendence could and should be achieved by members of the human species themselves (Huxley 1927, 195; Hauskeller 2012, 39). For Huxley, then, transhumanism was about access to fresh possibilities (Hauskeller 2012, 39).

Huxley strove to conceptually position human beings over and against animals in an essay entitled "The Uniqueness of Man" (1948). This uniqueness was exactly what, for Huxley, made eugenics possible and appropriate: "Man has the possibility of making [progress] the main feature of his own future evolution, and of guiding its course in relation to a deliberate aim" (28). Recall that this is also the argument of today's transhumanists Nick Bostrom and Anders Sandberg. Further, said Huxley, "[the human] must not be afraid of his own uniqueness . . . so far as our knowledge goes, human mind and personality are unique and constitute the highest product yet achieved by the cosmos. Let us not put off our responsibilities onto the shoulders of mythical gods or philosophical absolutes . . ." (1948, 28). So, for Huxley, evolutionary progress can be taken up as a tool, and should be taken up as a responsibility to the species. For him, superstitions regarding the importance of ceding to outside controls (playing God) should be put aside.

In another essay, "Eugenics and Society," Huxley ventures the following regarding the obligation to eugenics:

> Once the full implications of evolutionary biology are grasped, eugenics will inevitably become part of the religion of the future, or of whatever complex of sentiments may in the future take the place of organized religion. It is not merely a sane outlet for human altruism, but is of all outlets for altruism that which is most comprehensive and of the longest range. (1948, 28)

Notice that Huxley assumes full explanatory and progressive potential for evolutionary biology, meaning that harnessing that science allows us to take control of the future.

But, for Huxley, obstacles to the efficiency of eugenics must first be overcome if the eugenic ideal as future religion is to be realized (1948, 28). This meant that eugenics must be improved as a social science, a move which will improve its reputation (29). Along with an increasingly "careful" study of heritability (better genetics), eugenics must "use the results of this study for control" (32). He denounced Nazi Germany as precisely anti-eugenic because of its nationalism, which would subvert social eugenic goals by leading to "over-population and war" (55). Huxley believed that eugenicists must understand the social system and also must transform it at the risk of otherwise failing in scientific eugenic goals in the same way (33, 54, and 61). Ultimately, this essay represents an attempt to liberate eugenics from its bad reputation and from various biases, and align it with a renewed social outlook (33). For Huxley, eugenics is required because there is an "inherent tendency" of the gene pool to degrade over time—an idea, recall, later accepted by bioethicists Paul Ramsey (61). Here, for enhancement to be successful, the internal menace of bad genetics must be destroyed if humans are to bear up under menaces from without.

Generally, the importance of genetics alone, argued Huxley, should not be over *or* under-stated (1948, 41). As a factor, it was for him embedded among others in the scheme of evolutionary biology. Correlatively, Huxley's social goals involved more than genetic control. For example, although Huxley pushed for accessible birth control facilities and "family allowances, providing for sterilization here and financial relief for children there" (54), he also argued that environmental conditions like vitamins and food have greater impact than normally believed and that researches into twins prove that genetics was only one factor among many that should be controlled (37–38). He also explicitly denied the "genetic or eugenic significance of" "so-called racial traits" (39). Yet, he seems to mean merely that their significance has not *yet* been (eugenically) scientifically established. For example, he still believed it "wholly probable that true Negroes have a slightly lower average intelligence than the whites or yellows" (41). This idea supports his call for better genetics in order to avoid past mistakes in eugenic thinking.

Ultimately, despite his insistence on dethroning genetic factors, Huxley wanted to develop both social and genetic eugenic "patterns" that would improve the human being as a species. These could hold in "economic and communal life" and also "family and reproductive life" if group incentives were sought to make these patterns viable (1948, 55). Incentives could make it plausible for the individual to subordinate herself to the group (57). Control for her means enhancement for everyone (57). Huxley argued that birth control, by splitting reproductive and sexual functions, could help with this subordination of the individual to the group (58–59). The utopia of a future, better life appears to require undercutting existing lives, including the restriction of family-making and what may be referred to as human flourishing.

Bioethicists today note that the "shadow" of eugenics hangs over conversations regarding enhancement technologies and ask whether enhancement enthusiasm involves "new" or "old" eugenics (Buchanan *et al.* 2000, Crook 2008, Sparrow 2011). This leads some philosophers, like Huxley, to wonder in what sense eugenic policies *themselves*, wrested from the unjust practice of Nazi medicine, are morally wrong. Buchanan *et al.* argue that individual policies must be discussed without reference to the loaded eugenic label in order to allow history to guide the future (2000, 9–10). One point of consensus among these authors is the idea that some eugenic goals—for instance, better health for the population—become morally wrong when mixed with state coercion, but may not otherwise be wrong (Buchanan *et al.* 2000, 12–13). Bostrom is similarly concerned about state coercion. These authors also argue that eugenic goals become morally wrong when mixed with racist ideology and false biologically based race theories or other pseudosciences, but may not otherwise be wrong (27, 40–41). They note too that genetic determinism is a decisive element of the "shadow" of eugenics, a claim I pick up and deepen here at the close of the chapter (23–25).

Major elements of Huxley's post–Second World War rehabilitation of eugenics are still present, virtually unchanged, in bioethical conversation regarding the permissibility of human enhancement. Huxley felt the need to place the human uniquely within and among the evolution of species before arguing for the enhancement of human beings; today, we see that—for *both* proponents and opponents—the uniqueness of human nature (its inventiveness or its dignity, respectively) is still insisted upon (Engelhardt 1990; Habermas 2003; Fukuyama 2002; Kass 2002; Sandel 2004; Harris 2007, 2005b). For many today, as for Huxley in the mid-century, it is important to set aside individualism through medical, scientific, or other means in order to seek the greater good of the species. Altruism is important for these thinkers, including Julian Savulescu and Ingmar Persson, but they believe we cannot achieve altruism without bodily interventions and augmentations (2012).

Each of the moments I discuss in this chapter—the milieu of physical culture, the birth of the field of endocrinology, and postwar rehabilitation of eugenic strategies—is structurally linked with today's genetic visions of the human being. First, each moment showcases a reduction to the biological. Second, each moment defines what is desirable at least partly by what the desirable is not—the rejected body lurks in the background, a snarling threat to individuals and the social order. Finally, a utopian promise of a better life through physical interventions is made in each moment. One can grasp happiness, be more moral, be more responsible, be taller, be more intelligent, enjoy fertility, and enjoy one's children if only one exercises, takes vitamins, accepts a hormone supplement, or makes the right choice of marriage partner and child. A better, more moral, more beautiful and blissful life awaits you—and if you fail to choose this future, you do not deserve to enjoy it. Choosing to adjust one's body is positioned as key to happiness and control over one's future.

Further, enhancement strategies and transhumanism seem to depend on the elimination of difference—written as deviance—from the human community. Unless the deviant other is eliminated or enhanced, individual enhancement is under threat. The transhumanist enhancer believes that there is a right to happiness (bliss), and that unless an entire *community* of enhanced persons (normal, abled persons) exists my enjoyment of this state will be stymied. One's individual happiness and freedom will be blocked by the Roma (Wiggam), the short (Wells), or the deviant public who know nothing of the laws of inheritance and lack birth control (Huxley, the first transhumanist). This is a perverse reversal of the feminist claim regarding the relationality of persons; biopower teaches us that I cannot be excellent unless everyone is.[5]

GENETIC VISIONS

I turn now to consider genetic determinism, the most recent variety of biological reduction, and its connection to enhancement and transhumanism. Genetic determinism underlies today's debates over enhancement and matches the reduction of social problems to biological explanations in the past 100 years of enhancement thinking. Biological reductions structure interplays between deviance and normality. Many bioethicists and philosophers critique the notion of a genetic telos (Buchanan *et al.* 2000, 85; Brock 1992; Klitzman 2012; Nelkin and Lindee 1995; Siever 1997). Evelyn Fox Keller gives an exceptional philosophical history of what she calls the genetic century—the twentieth—and suggests that the era will be superseded by the dominance of other constructs (2000; cf. McNally and Glasner 2007). She argues that genetic research actually demonstrates that the gene is not the primary unit of heredity; yet oversimplifications abound, especially because they are practical for researchers in attracting money and attention (Radick 2001). For her, understanding units within a system (the gene) is less valuable than tracing the dynamism of a system (the organism) itself; in future we will need better vocabulary to describe the movement of biological heredity. But, as Keller realizes, the mid-century discovery of the structure of the double-helix, paired with the interpretation of the gene as a set of specific instructions (the "central dogma" of genetic determinism), still has unabated influence. This influence extends to debate over human enhancement, along with discussion regarding individual traits.

The genetic vision of the human being is entrenched, especially as a result of the Human Genome Project and the international scientific community's continued work under that banner. Popular discourse treats genotype as the directive fundamental core of the human being, and so, if we want to improve the human condition, genotype is considered the place to begin. Nobel Prize winner James Watson, whose research team first modeled DNA in 1953, is vocally in favor of utilizing genetic research in hope of radical human transformation. Watson advocates screening strategies and eugenics. In 1998 he infamously remarked:

> I think it's complete nonsense . . . saying we're sacred and should not be changed . . . Evolution can be just damn cruel, and to say we've got a perfect genome and there's some sanctity? I'd like to know where that idea comes from because it's utter silliness . . . To try to give it any more meaning than it deserves in some quasi-mystical way is for Steven Spielberg or somebody like that. It's just plain aura, up in the sky—I mean, it's crap. (Brave 2003)

Watson rejects the idea of sanctity of life when deployed as a reason for not interfering with the human genome, which he claims is the source of human suffering because it has not been improved upon. He rejects ratcheting up the meaning of genome into a benevolent god.

Notably, Watson's critique of enshrining the genome is shared in the reflections of disability scholars and bioethicists who also critique views rooted in genetic determinism (e.g. Scully 2008). But, the critique should yield a different conclusion from Watson's; that is, an alternative to the idea that faulty genetics should be seen as such and transformed via eugenics to end suffering. Watson's conclusion shores up the importance of the genotype in daily life by claiming that it is an important site for intervention. Instead, one could conclude that the importance of genotype is overstated, and suggest other shared projects of "enhancement" that focus on social and political transformation through social and political change, not biological change.

Yet genetic variations, considered defects, are today thought to constitute a wrongful birth or wrongful life (Buchanan *et al.* 2000; Roberts 2009; Rogers 1999; Savulescu 2008; Shiffrin 1999; cf. Ramsey 1970). At the very least, a-typical genetic structure is thought to trouble the decision to conceive or to continue with an existing pregnancy (cf. Parens and Asch 2000). Many bioethicists accept as a fundamental premise the idea that the avoidance of disabilities or diseases through genetic means is desirable. Indeed, at the extreme, they also argue that it is immoral to fail to avoid disability or diseases (Boyle and Savulescu 2003; Buchanan *et al.* 2000, e.g. 100–101; Savulescu 2001b and 2008; Rogers 1999). In fact, transhumanists take for granted that genetic improvement via selection (thus avoiding wrongful birth and wrongful life) would provide human beings with greater freedom and multiply choice—thereby providing access to an enhanced life of great happiness and well-being.

These ideas are as old as bioethics itself; forty years ago, Ramsey concluded that it is consistent with both the genetic and religious visions of humanity to believe that serious genetic defects should preclude procreation (1970, 43–44). He worried about the proliferation of "hideous birth defects" and "monstrosities" and argued that a Christian ethic could, ironically, require parents to exercise precautions against having children when they are the carriers of certain traits (8, 57–59). He held this despite the fact that he felt that genetic interventions constituted playing God and should be avoided. In other words, the desire to avoid genetic deviation is strong enough to overthrow the "playing God" objection for a Christian bioethicist.

Proposed means for the avoidance of disability and the pursuit of enhancement are often rendered much the same if not identical (Savulescu 2001a). That is, positive and negative eugenics are twinned in bioethics. Bioethicists have argued that it makes sense to accept many different kinds of human enhancements, because of the deep similarity between reasons for avoiding negative states and reasons for pursuing positive ones (e.g. Harris 2011, 147). Along these lines, Peter Singer writes:

> Many people say that they accept selection against serious diseases and disabilities, but not for enhancement beyond what is normal. There is, however, no bright line between selection against disabilities and selection for positive

> characteristics. From selecting against Huntington's Disease it is no great step to selecting against genes that carry a significantly elevated risk of breast or colon cancer, and from there it is easy to move to giving one's child a better than average genetic health profile. (2011, 278)

Singer uses the above, what he considers morally approvable actions undertaken to avoid disability or disease states, against Michael Sandel's argument that enhancement erodes a sense of life's giftedness (2004). He claims that there must be limits on this idea, since even Sandel does not argue against

> current practices of prenatal diagnosis that are aimed at eliminating serious genetic disease and disabilities. The argument for taking life as a gift clearly has limits. If it is outweighed by the importance of avoiding children with serious diseases or disabilities, it may also be outweighed by the positive characteristics that genetic selection can bring. (2009, p. 279)

Acceptance of the pursuit of enhancement, in other words, conceptually and rhetorically relies the rejection of the deviant body—as throughout the last century of enhancement thinking (cf. Parens 1995, 142).

The genetic conception of the human being can be viewed as the ground of "genetic essentialism" or genetic determinism (Scully 2008, Nelkin and Lindee 1995, 38–49). Some decry the resulting "gene-mania" which "encourage[s] unrealistic hopes for genetic solutions to all sorts of problems" (Buchanan *et al.* 2000, 23, 24–25).[6] I here describe genetic determinism and discuss the fact that central figures (even those who self-consciously disavow it or, like Buchanan *et al.*, warn of the support genetic determinism lends to eugenics) who advocate for various kinds of enhancements still operate by giving credence to genetic determinism—especially by presuming that genotype can produce a predictable set of results and is susceptible to manipulation through pure "choice" and no "chance" (Buchanan *et al.* 2000, 24–25; Glover 1984, 2006; Oliver 2010). Genetic determinism increases stigma connected to disability and impairment and aids in reductive thinking that ignores the social and cultural factors which in turn frame and constitute disability.

Genetic Determinism

Genetic determinism is a view about causes which assumes the sole or primary importance of genetic factors in individual outcome (for persons—i.e., with regard to phenotype, complex behaviors, and other traits). Often this view involves valuing gene action as autonomous cause or giving undue priority to genetic explanations over environmental or diverse multifactorial explanations (Buchanan *et al.* 2000, 23–24; Lippman 1991 and 1993; Lotz 2008; Nelkin and Lindee 1995, 2). Most scientists, especially geneticists, condemn genetic determinism as false or incorrect, and therefore scientific or philosophical beliefs and assertions that stem from it are considered highly problematic (e.g. de Melo-Martín 2005, 526; Sober 2000). Bioethicists, as aforementioned, often take care to explicitly reject genetic determinism (e.g. Buchanan *et al.* 2000, 24–25; de Melo-Martín 2005, 527; Scully 2008, e.g. 5–6). Yet, mistaken beliefs supporting genetic determinism still have an impact on bioethics, medicine, and conceptions of disability; for example, genetic determinism and related ideas support a strict binary between norm and deviance that variation in the human genome belies (Scully 2008, 24; cf. discussion of normalization in Tremain 2006). This is especially true of trans-humanist discussion of enhancement technologies, which often assumes that genetic enhancements can open up a better and a more just future. Genetic determinism, by far not the best argument regarding gene action, is unfortunately influential in academic, political, and social registers and so deserves careful attention.

The assumed explanatory power of genes and the particular cases cited in the media often encourage expanding what has been called the "one gene—one disease" concept, or the OGOD concept, to proliferating features and traits that parents and the public consider unwanted or wanted (Dar-Nimrod and Heine 2010, 12; cf. Conrad 1997 and 2002). Only some outcomes are indicated by a single gene; "monogenic" conditions are relatively rare (an example is cystic fibrosis), and most relationships between genes and outcomes are quite complicated and mediated heavily by unpredictable or yet to be understood factors (Dar-Nimrod and Heine 2010, 13). Many phenotypic outcomes are multifactorial; this means that more than one gene impacts the phenotype of the individual. But, phenotypic outcomes are also the result of genes, environment, and individual behaviors working together. Despite the fact that the OGOD concept expresses the exception—not the rule—of genetic causation, it is the basic picture of gene action as portrayed in popular media and that most often endorsed among laypersons (Dar-Nimrod and Heine 2010, 4; Nelkin and Lindee 1995). The problem isn't that "reductive" genetic explanations are *never* appropriate, but rather that the way reductive explanations are popularized and widely applied is problematic (Scully 2008, 6). Genetic determinism and the expansion of the OGOD concept, at the very least, obfuscate accurate explanations of causality.

Relatedly, screening procedures for particular outcomes, even when "isolated," are highly complex and uncertain. For example, the breast cancer 1 (BRCA1) and breast cancer 2 (BRCA2) genes are associated with hereditary ovarian and breast cancers. But, over 200 different mutations on these two genes have been described, and little is known about how context—both biological and environmental—impacts the relevance of these mutations (de Melo-Martín 2005, 528). Furthermore, the BRCA1 and BRCA2 genes are only associated with a small slice of breast and ovarian cancers—between 5 and 10 percent (Dar-Nimrod and Heine 2010, 13; de Melo-Martín 2005, 528). In the context of the venture capitalism of genetic testing, touting the screening of these genes as a test "for" breast cancer is misleading. Meanwhile, available direct-to-consumer screening for the "FTO" (fat mass and obesity associated) gene has been scrutinized for its "futility" and failure to contextualize genetic information into dynamic gene-behavior relationships (Veerman 2011). According to JL Veerman, screening for the FTO gene has very little predictive power, does not add information about propensity to disease, and distracts attention away from more efficacious health measures (Veerman 2011; see also Kolata 2012).

It is easy to blame sensational media headlines for the OGOD problem. For decades, news reports have heralded "The Gay Gene," "The Evolution Gene," and genes for obsessive-compulsive disorder, among other conditions (Dar-Nimrod and Heine 2010, 13; Nelkin and Lindee 1995, 93). Popular books even describe the gene in agential and even immortal terms, for example, "The Selfish Gene" (Nelkin and Lindee 1995, 53). But, responsibility for the ubiquity of OGOD, and therefore support for genetic determinism, does not belong to the media alone. The necessity of fundraising and attracting exciting coverage for those in the scientific community means scientists over-promise the explanatory potential of genetic research (Nelkin and Lindee 1995, 5–7). Popular media often echo the language of the scientific studies they report. Descriptions of genetic action as deterministic structure attention-grabbing and money-generating narratives (Nelkin and Lindee 1995).

Moving forward, it is important to keep in mind that the presence of genes does not necessarily mean that those genes will be expressed. Incomplete penetrance and variable expressivity mean that persons with the same genotype can differ in phenotype. Gene penetrance is a statistical measure of the expression of a gene among individuals (70 percent penetrance, for example, indicates that 7 of every 10 people with a particular genotype express the associated phenotype). Variable expressivity, meanwhile, can be explained using *polydactyly* as an example. Polydactyly is a heritable condition may result in extra toes or extra fingers. Polydactyly may "penetrate" (i.e., what we call polydactyly might be phenotypically apparent) but is variably expressive (Miko 2008). To return to my earlier example of hereditary breast and ovarian cancers, de Melo-Martín notes that rates of expressivity for the BRCA1 and BRCA2 genes in different contexts is unknown and varies among the 200 different mutations. This makes risk assessment difficult; mutations on either of these genes does not mean that one will get cancer (2005, 528).[7] So-called genetic susceptibility must be contextualized by behavior, environment, and other factors (Lewontin 1992, 30). There is a distinction between strong genetic explanations (OGOD explanations) and weak genetic explanations (Dar-Nimrod and Heine 2010, 4–5). Again, the vast majority of genetic explanations are "weak"—that is, they describe genes as "altering risk assessments, modifying susceptibilities, [and] changing probabilities" (4). Weak genetic explanations can be entered into a set of assessments regarding risk that are far from deterministic. Yet, risk assessment is what most presume genetics does best.

So far, I have discussed the causal complications which make strong genetic determinism fallacious. I described genetic determinism as a mistaken view about causes. But, the genetic reduction involved in a picture of gene action informed by genetic determinism has influence that goes *beyond* questions of causality, and simply correcting and adjusting popular understanding of gene action will not banish the ethical and political problems associated with a strong focus on or preference for genetic explanations. In fact, this more complex understanding of gene action does not banish scientific problems, either. According to bioethicist Immaculada de Melo-Martín, focusing on "interactionist" variables, "far from debunking genetic determinism, simply reinforces it, because genes are still represented as containing information about how the organism will develop" (2005, 526). So, it is important to expand our discussion beyond looking for a better or more accurate portrait of causality.

Genetic determinism supports insidious 1) *essentialism* and 2) *naturalization* of socially defined and constructed categories of persons, such as those defined by sexual orientation, race, gender, and disability. In other words, genetic determinism is a biological reduction. Related essentialism and naturalization work together in a way that increases stigma (and therefore social alienation) and disguises the social and cultural factors that impact definitions of disease and disability.

I turn first to essentialism and its connection to genetic determinism, taking cues from philosophers of disability and survey research conducted in the field of social psychology. Bioethicist and geneticist Jackie Scully links genetic reduction to essentialism. She orients genetic determinism as one variety of biological reduction, and describes it as the view that "DNA sequences" "encode instructions for proteins" which "determine" traits and health (2008, 5). She argues that reductive explanations of traits and behaviors that rely merely on DNA sequences establish a mistaken belief that there is a "canonical" human genotype, which is the blueprint for normal persons. Any deviations (mutations, deletions, additions) from this canonical genotype are treated as abnormalities (2008, 6). Yet, Scully notes, there is no such blueprint—variation in human genotype is constant, and a strict and meaningful binary between normal and abnormal is simply not supported by genetic science. The importance accorded genetic "normalcy" is excessive; indeed, the newest chromosomal microarray tests intended for use by potential parents indicate merely that a genome is "abnormal," that is, that it deviates from the genome of a presumed healthy person, but not what deviation means.

Chromosomal microarray is said to be more reliable than karyotyping (visual screening) in detecting fetal abnormality. This method detects abnormalities in 1 out of every 60 pregnancies in which karyotyping identified the fetus as "normal." Chromosomal microarray directly compares fetal DNA to DNA from a presumptively "healthy person" to identify genetic deviations (Wapner *et al.* 2012; Fitzgerald 2012). The chromosomal microarray method thus assumes a human genetic blueprint—that is, a normal genotype, deviance from which is risky and open to medical diagnosis.

Genetic determinism has a strong psychological hold and operates much like essentialist thinking operates. Social psychologists Ilan Dar-Nimrod and Steven Heine demonstrate that the gene serves as an "essence placeholder"; specifically, genetic determinism maps onto the essentialist thinking (2010, 2). Those surveyed by Dar-Nimrod and Heine had a tendency to presume an underlying essence unique to social categories and groups, yet this essence remained "abstract" and "undefined" (e.g. the essence of a cat, a person, an African-American person, a woman, a disabled person) (2). Dar-Nimrod and Heine identify the elements of an essence in terms of its "causal relationship between essence and expected characteristics," its "stability," and that it is "presumed to be immutable" (2). The gene is a convenient and metaphorically rich place-holder for already-presumed yet abstract essences and carries forward the causal, immutable, and stable properties thought natural to an essence (see also similar work in social psychology regarding essentialism and genetic bias: Haslam 2011; Keller 2005).

I turn now to naturalization. Again, this is the term I use to refer to the transformation of dynamic and historically contingent medical, social, and political categories and concepts into supposedly naturally occurring facts about the body. Genetic determinist views see dynamic characteristics, behaviors, and socially constructed traits through the presumed explanatory power of genes, thus naturalizing them and removing them from relevant contexts. If there is a "gay gene," for example, that transforms queer identities into a biological fact; this strategic essentialism carries its own risks (Byrd and Hughey 2015; Walters 2014).[8] The political nuances of identity formation, the public and private pressures which have, created a system of being "out" or "closeted," and historical and geographical contexts of the meaning of queer identities is hidden via naturalization. Similarly, the political and social nuances of personal identification as or medical diagnosis of Asperger syndrome and autism are lost if these conditions are considered essential or genetically determined properties of bodies.

The recent decision of the editors of the DSM-V (the latest edition of the *Diagnostic and Statistical Manual of Mental Disorders*) to shift Asperger syndrome onto the autism spectrum and cease to recognize it as a discrete category should showcase how important historically contextual diagnostic decisions can be with regard to disability ("Asperger's" 2012). In a memoir, John Elder Robison gave an account of how important the label of "Asperger's" was to him as he constructed a disability identity (2008). Now, politically active "Aspies" find themselves rendered invisible by the very medical categorization schemes that previously served to (problematically) socially define them, and are newly considered autistic (a fact which will change prevalence statistics). Meanwhile, the United States Center for Disease Control revisited estimations of the prevalence of autism based on telephone surveys and new criteria, suggesting that 1 in 50 children are affected (Heasley 2013). Another example of the importance of historical and political context to the question of disability and its construction is the category of learning disabilities and the diagnostic and statistical blossoming of a variety of these conditions as public educational strategies and policies change.

As philosopher of disability and Foucauldian Shelley Tremain puts it in a discussion of prenatal testing and screening procedures, naturalization can also be described as a problem of *materialization*; that is, the hypostatization of discursive categories into "real" categories (2006, 39). Similarly, the strategic analogy made by disability activists between sex/gender and impairment/disability in order to support disability rights campaigns for equal protection under the law problematically treats impairment (separated from disability) as natural or uninfluenced by medical, political, legal, and social forces. Tremain therefore interrogates the category of "fetal impairment" and seeks to deflate its status as a "real" category or a "natural kind" (Tremain 2006, 39 and 49; see also Tremain 2001, 2002). Ultimately, even if perfect genetic science were available, we would not have full "knowledge" of disability, because disability is a social and discursive category that bears upon bodies.

Bioethics and Genetic Determinism

Popular media does contribute to mistaken beliefs supporting genetic determinism, especially when reporting scientific findings and research plans regarding genetics. But, these findings and plans are often presented by scientists themselves in ways that problematically describe gene action. This is one issue bioethicists should attend to and work against. According to de Melo-Martín, bioethicists should also attend to an issue that penetrates a level deeper; that of communication about genetics within the field of bioethics itself. She argues that bioethicists make significant mistakes when making moral arguments which contribute to false beliefs among readers about gene action and in turn support genetic determinism (2005). She identifies citing unrepresentative cases (such as OGOD cases or traits that are autosomal dominant, like Huntington's disease) when discussing reproductive technology as one such mistake (527).

Another mistake is to use simplified cases, as in the case of discussing the ethical ramifications of genetic testing "when information about diseases with a genetic component and the predictably of genetic tests for these diseases is presented in simplistic ways" (de Melo-Martín 2005, 528). I already mentioned the misleading discussion around BRCA1 and BRCA2 screening; de Melo-Martín also refers to genetic testing for Alzheimer's disease as a case that is often represented simplistically (528).

But, complex beliefs related to genetic determinism are an even more significant problem in the field of bioethics than de Melo-Martín outlines. Genetic determinism poses threats within bioethics beyond threats precipitated by miscommunications between experts and laypersons, bioethicists and readers. Genetic determinism strongly influences philosophical discussion in bioethics regarding genetic screening, genetic selection of embryos, genetic enhancement, and transhumanist desires for enhanced genetic futures. In fact, philosophical views promulgated by bioethicists on these topics appear rooted in genetic determinism. Genetic determinism therefore shapes significant arguments in bioethics, and is more than a mere regrettable byproduct of some modes of discussion. This situation holds despite the fact that "practically every geneticist alive" and plenty of bioethicists reject genetic determinism (de Melo-Martín 2005, 526).

Genetic determinism affects bioethics as a field by delimiting advances in ethical thinking or obscuring important scientific knowledge and significantly contributes to the twinned force of stigma and synecdoche—the tendency to take a part as representative of the whole. Many recognize that mistakes supporting genetic determinism in the media and in communicative efforts with laypersons should be combated. But, the problem runs deeper than that; it is time to recognize how entrenched genetic and other biological reductions are in discussions of enhancement and disability and, therefore, in discussions of illness and health.

CONCLUSION

To deepen understanding regarding transhumanism and today's general bioethical conversation regarding enhancement, I investigated its ancestry through a discussion of key moments in the past century of enhancement thinking. While I did not seek to uncover a telos or a metaphysical truth, I hoped to uncover the ways enhancement thinking has been written onto the body. The alternative eugenic history I traced allowed me to point to and track locations of biopower, including: the reduction of human life, morality, and meaning to the level of the biological or the physical; the rejection of the deviant body; and the lasting romantic, utopian thinking undergirding the quest for enhancement, even as that quest grew and changed. Just as in the case of transhumanism today, justifications of enhancement strategies in the twentieth century operated by responding to and exploiting desires to increase happiness, freedom, and choice, and at the same time played upon fears of deviant others who would threaten one's own health and the health of the population and nation.

Biological reductions make it plausible to view the discipline of the body, along with choosing health (the right marriage partner, or diet, exercise, and hormone supplements), as a route to happiness and bliss. In other words, physical and mental health, and importantly choice-making, were equated with morality, happiness, and sociability; the primary operating assumption is that the body is the site for any intervention aimed toward improving human life. This puts to the side any discussion regarding political and social impacts on the construction or maintenance of health and sickness, disability and ability. Disability and deviance are continually referenced and reconstructed as a variety of ways to understand health go in and out of vogue. Rejected bodies are repeatedly painted as too dependent or as irresponsible and dangerous (sickness as sin; weakness as crime) in order to justify their exclusion or even their extermination through sterilization or other means. They have failed to choose health—they are not responsible choice-makers—and therefore their deviance must be rejected as a menace to the health of the community. From the Roma identified by Wiggam to short individuals threatening the primacy of the tall in the imagination of H. G. Wells, the deviant body is seen not only as an outlier, but an "other" with the ability to preclude the possibility of the norm's flourishing. In a perverse reversal of feminist theories of relationality, everyone must enhance—the community itself must be normalized—for individual enhancement to occur.

Today, just as in the heyday of physical culture, the immorality and irresponsibility of sickness and weakness shapes the public imaginary and belief in the heritability of *moral* traits and *social* happiness appears in bioethical debates over enhancement. Central to all of this, then, is a double-edged weapon for use against persons positioned as disabled or experiencing disability: either disability can and therefore should be overcome through medical or non-medical discipline, or disability must be removed from the general population by way of segregation so as to dissipate the threat to health and freedom of the population. Disabled lives are not worth living, and if they cannot be transformed, they must be rejected—or, perhaps, disallowed from the beginning through selection and screening. Meanwhile, certain bodies are valorized as free and healthy in opposition to the disabled body, while a cost—benefit analysis of the value of expending resources on rejected lives becomes intelligible. These largely unexamined assumptions are still operative, and the supposedly obvious claim that disability is undesirable is used to cut off questions regarding the desirability of enhancement.

Transhumanism is rooted in the rejection of deviant embodiment; the view repeats the biological reductions necessary to support both the destructive belief that morality and appropriate sociability increase and decrease along with physical fitness and mental acuity and the attempt to solve social problems through intervention upon the body. Transhumanists make the body central to problem-solving while at the same time endeavoring to transcend it completely, rejecting embodiment in its entirety. While enhancement once focused on the discipline of the body and its perfection through technology, as in "physical culture" at the turn of the twentieth century, enhancement in the twenty-first century promoted by transhumanism is focused on leaving the body behind altogether.

This move is not limited to academic circles; popular internet discourse concerning human enhancement often expresses a hatred or disgust for fleshly embodiment. In response to an article entitled "How to Build the Perfect Human" on popular futuristic website i09, which suggested splicing animal traits in order to gain their capabilities (Ingus-Arkell 2012); a commentator wrote: "To make a better human, I'd scrap the protein and meat altogether" (Feb 15, 2012). A posthuman will transcend the neediness and vulnerability of the flesh, trading up to replaceable and strong non-organic parts. Futurist and Google executive Ray Kurzweil argues that soon sex will be virtual, and if we are unfortunate enough to have sex with a fleshly partner we can take comfort in a techno-overlay which will project the image of a desired individual or celebrity upon that partner (Kurzweil and Grossman 2010, 96). Sex is not desirable unless we can have sex in the realm of wishes and fantasy:

> virtual sex will be better in some ways and certainly safer. Virtual sex will provide sensations that are more intense and pleasurable than conventional sex, as well as physical experiences that currently do not exist. Virtual sex is also the ultimate in safe sex, as there is no risk of pregnancy or transmission of disease. (2000, 747)

Kurzweil rejects the body as limiting pleasure and as the site of risk. The transhumanist discussion, both popular and academic, is consistent with rhetoric used throughout the past century of enhancement thinking, but additionally rejects embodiment completely.

In the next chapter, I explore a key aspect of the contemporary transhuman fantasy—the child of choice, for whom freedom and happiness are unlocked. I consider Julian Savulescu's claim regarding a moral obligation to create the best children possible—an enhancement strategy rooted in genetic selection. This idea coheres with the notion of the "right to an open future"—a bundle of rights thought to ensure future autonomy—and genetic harm or wrongful birth (Feinberg 1980; cf. Mills 2003).[9] The aims of procreative beneficence again call to mind Snyder and Mitchell's critique of the utopian eugenic vision of a world without bodies, uncontaminated by deviance and needs. This promise is the backdrop of the genetic obligation to provide future children with increased health and maximized choice. I will consider the "impaired fetus," diagnosable in the womb, as the threatening and rejectable body (Tremain 2006). Objections to genetic selection from disability theorists, along with the Foucauldian framework I have been employing, can help us understand what is objectionable about valorizing the abled body in the arena of reproductive technology.

NOTES

1. This is the term I use to refer to the transformation of dynamic and historically contingent medical, social, and political categories and concepts into supposedly naturally occurring, transhistorical and transcultural facts about the body (see Tremain 2001, 2002, 2006; Wendell 1996 on the naturalization of disability, for example).
2. For an excellent treatment of the hyper-sexualization of women with disabilities and their treatment as irresponsible and overly fertile, see Snyder and Mitchell 2006, 86.
3. For treatment of the frequent conflation between being disabled and irresponsibility (specifically with regard to labor), see Frank 2000, 71. See also Nancy Fraser and Linda Gordon's genealogical investigation of "dependency" in the United States and its nuances with regard to debates over the provision of welfare (1994).
4. Aldous Huxley's work is often referenced in bioethical discussions about enhancement. Bioethicist Leon Kass, who served on George W. Bush's presidential bioethics council, uses Aldous Huxley's dystopian novel *A Brave New World* as an example of a dystopia brought about through technological interventions on the natural (2002). Aldous Huxley is also the author of *After Many a Summer Dies the Swan* (originally published in 1939), which deals with an aging man's search for immortality. Yet, Julian Huxley, Aldous' brother, was also a writer and a social philosopher.
5. My thanks to Lisa Guenther for articulating this insightful point.
6. Despite their attention to fallacies regarding genetic causation and the inclusion of an appendix on the topic by Elliott Sober, Buchanan *et al.* still indulge in a genetically based version of identity without justifying its aptness (2000, 85).
7. Any testing or screening procedure is susceptible to false positives and false negatives.
8. Earlier categorization in the *Diagnostic and Statistical Manual of Mental Disorders* of queer identity as pathological was eventually dropped in part due to the strategic essentialism strategies employed by gay activists, culminating in 1973 (Nelkin and Lindee 1995, 120–121).
9. Savulescu is a utilitarian, and therefore does not explicitly use the notion of rights. But, I will show that his reasoning is continuous with the concept of the right to an open future.

Chapter 4

Choosing, for Choice's Sake

A Case Study

While enhancement often conjures up images of superhero strength, or Ray Kurzweil's and Randal Koene's suggestion that humans "upload" their thoughts and Nick Bostrom's suggestion that grey matter be "copied" in silicon, the transhumanist strategy of genetic selection is just as important for transhumanist visions of the future (see Savulescu 2001, 2008, and Kahane 2009; for supporting ideas among more mainstream bioethicists, see Buchanan *et al.* 2000; Liao *et al.* 2012). Julian Savulescu's proposed moral duty of procreative beneficence, a strong version of reproductive responsibility, is a prominent example of this strategy (2001b, 2008). Procreative beneficence urges those considering reproduction to apply evolving genetic technologies as they are developed to create the "best" child with the greatest future options. Transhumanism, here, would preclude the existence of particular individuals based on genetic profiles taken before birth. This is, perhaps, the first step of the total rejection of the body—that is, carrying out a consistent and (it is believed) "justifiable rejection" of the "defective" fetus (Saxton 2000, 158). The enhancement strategy of genetic selection asks and answers the biopolitical question "who will live?" even as it appears to provide parents with new options. Genetic selection is framed in bioethics discussions as the choice of particular, "better" embryos or fetuses which can lead to the enhancement of quality of life for those who are living and ensure the shared resource of an enhanced genetic pool for future generations. In this chapter, I bring transhumanist utopian thinking into sharp focus by treating negative genetic selection as a case study.

Genetic selection can refer to a host of activities surrounding reproductive decision-making. The roughest distinction often made among these activities is between positive and negative genetic selection, that is, genetic selection for particular traits or against particular traits. I maintain this distinction here for the sake of clarity and responding to the work of others, although it problematically resonates with negative evaluations of disability traits. Genetic selection can also be said to occur through the choice of a partner with whom one might reproduce, or the timing of a pregnancy, insofar as both of these things impact the genotype of the fetus and the eventual child. But, this is not the sense in which I use it here. Negative genetic selection can be achieved through the choice of one embryo rather than another for implantation or through the termination of a pregnancy upon the discovery of a particular trait, genetic markers, or genetic susceptibility by way of screening practices. Medical professionals advise women to undergo these procedures at different times before and during pregnancy.

Preimplantation diagnosis combined with invitro fertilization allows potential parents to test embryos for markers and indications of both disease and non-disease traits (a common distinction) prior to implantation. This testing can lead to the decision of which embryo to implant, or, perhaps, to implant no embryo at all. Prior, even, to that early stage, potential parents can undergo their own set of genetic tests to determine probabilities for carrying forward traits or the risk of certain conditions to future children. Finally, prenatal genetic testing can be carried out after a pregnancy is initiated. For example, amniocentesis can be conducted after a woman becomes pregnant and can lead to the termination of the pregnancy if the parent so chooses. The same is true of maternal serum screening, testing via ultrasound and chorionic villus sampling (CVS) (Parens and Asch 2000, 45–7; Davis 2010, 2). New tests are continually being developed. Recently a new test for Down syndrome was announced, called MaterniT21. This test can be used at 10 weeks into pregnancy and, unlike its predecessor, amniocentesis, does not increase the risk of miscarriage. It tests a blood sample taken from the mother's arm (Hill 2012). Additionally, as discussed in Chapter 3, new chromosomal microarray testing procedures—said to be better than karyotyping at detecting "fetal abnormality"—are now available. Chromosomal microarray compares fetal DNA and DNA from a presumed "healthy person" to identify genetic deviations. This practice of identifying deviation from a clearly arbitrary "normal" genotype is a suspect and stigmatizing practice that feeds into confusion about the meaning of testing.

In this discussion, I treat these various screening procedures as significantly similar. Any screening procedure undertaken to assess the health of a potential child can lead potential parents to a choice discursively constructed in bioethics literature and practically constructed by the current medical climate: that is, the choice of whether to bring a particular fetus to term after it is diagnosed or named.

Negative genetic selection occurs regularly in the United States; for example, 19 studies conducted in 1988 show that 87 percent of fetuses which tested positive for Trisomy 21 (indicating Down syndrome) were aborted (Mansfield *et al.* 1999, 810). Recent estimates place this number above 90 percent (James 2009). Popular discourse situates Down syndrome as a risk best avoided at any cost. But, to frame indications for Down syndrome, among other genetic indications, as risky support genetic bias and the untenable belief that a body "marked" with a particular trait reliably enjoys a lessened quality of life in comparison to an unmarked body specifically because of genotype. The logic of genetic selection relies on naturalized and materialized versions of disability that ignore their discursive, historical, and social settings.

For example, genetic markers for Down syndrome indicate a wide range of potential phenotypic characteristics, the meaning of which depend on reception in society, but genetic indications of Down syndrome are often represented as all-or-nothing affairs that reveal a "Down's baby" whose quality of life will be low. The practice of genetic selection participates in an unjust hierarchy of value which in turn hides the social and political forces which construct it in the first place. As Shelley Tremain puts it, "in terms of this conception of risks in pregnancy . . . an increasing number of variations between humans are attributed to allegedly prediscursive genetic structures" (2006, 47). A systematic disregard for stigmatizing and unjust discursive, political, and social conditions and factors feeds and is fed by an over-emphasis on genetic factors.

When one seeks to critique genetic selection against fetuses symbolically structured as disabled, a conflict surfaces between feminist convictions regarding "choice" as it is commonly understood in a reproductive context and the justice claims forwarded by disability activists who see societal endorsement of genetic selection as akin to eugenics (Morris 1991). Feminist Judy Rohrer writes: "The intersection of 'choice' with the valuation of a disabled life provokes a clash that rocks our rhetoric and takes us back into active theorizing about *whose humanity is supported and valued and under what circumstances*" (2005, 58, emphasis mine). In order to accomplish this active theorizing, awake to systematic oppression, feminist disability theorists must meet transhumanists and other bioethicists head-on regarding negative selection and refuse the co-option of the language of "choice." Ableism is linked tightly to "marked bodies" of all kinds and the reasoning of sexism, racism, classism, and heteronormativity, all of which rely on a stigmatized other whose difference is often rendered as biological (Mitchell and Snyder 2000, ix). The worry that a critique of negative genetic selection may be anti-choice in the reproductive sense drives an unnecessary wedge between feminist theorists and disability theorists and obscures the ways in which ableism and sexism are fused together. Feminist advocates of disability rights and feminist thinkers should not be forced to walk a tightrope between supposedly competing interests on this issue. In what follows, I launch a multifaceted critique of genetic selection, which borrows from the disability critique articulated by Adrienne Asch, and demonstrate that such a critique is consistent with and even enhances reproductive justice. At the end of the chapter, using the issue of negative genetic selection as a backdrop, I call the purported alignment and political alliance some see between transhumanists and persons with disabilities into question.

PROCREATIVE BENEFICENCE

Transhumanist thinker Julian Savulescu argues that that "eugenic" genetic selection is the best way to achieve human enhancement—for him, it is superior to genetic engineering (with Hemsley *et al.* 2006). His principle of procreative beneficence requires that parents use any available technology to pursue the creation of the best child possible (2001b, 414). He frames this as a parental moral duty to ensure children have the best chance at the best life. For him, this moral obligation means that parents should do what they have the most reason to do in response to testing results (415). For example, when engaging in preimplantation genetic diagnosis, absent any other overriding reasons for choosing a particular embryo (I will return to this in a moment), the parent should choose the embryo with the best chances for the best life (416–417). For him, reproduction is like "playing the Wheel of Fortune. You should use all available information and choose the option must likely to bring about the best outcome" (414). Notice the rhetorical juxtaposition of parents as rational choice-makers up against a game of chance; in this scheme, genetic information is framed as reliable information in a sea of uncertainty.

Savulescu defines the best life as "the life of the most well-being" (2001b, 419). For Savulescu, *intelligence* and *memory* are multipurpose and can always enhance one's quality of life, no matter what one's individual goals, so these traits should be maximized where possible (420). These traits are multipurpose because, he argues, on any theory of well-being (he gives three examples: "hedonistic," "desire-fulfillment" and "objective list" theories), capacities such as "choosing means to satisfy ends," and "imagining alternative pleasures" are important (419–421). One must be able to make social connections and absorb information about the world, activities Savulescu believes are augmented by individual intelligence, and, ultimately, predictable through genetic testing. Savulescu's goal of heightened well-being is the justification for the use of screening and selection practices and the moral obligation to abide by the principle of procreative beneficence. The underlying assumption is that genotype is the appropriate vector for augmenting quality of life and seeking the best life.

Genetic markers linked with disability are among the traits he targets as worse. He claims it is morally conscientious to select against these traits (Savulescu 2008). For example, he uses the rubella case; a woman with rubella could have a child now and risk them being deaf and blind, but could also wait three months and have a healthy child. According to procreative beneficence, even though no one is "harmed" by these cases, because the child in question would not otherwise exist (see Parfit 1984 on the non-identity problem), it is still better to wait. This is because we should initiate a pregnancy under circumstances which ensure the best chance at the best life, and conceiving when one has rubella does not fulfill this (2001b, 417–418). This means that disability and disease are marked out by Savulescu as interrupting the best chance at the best life.

Savulescu further argues that one must also select against any other genes that might obstruct the good life, like a "bad temper" or "asthma" (2001b, 414–15, cf. 2001a). According to Savulescu, any trait can impact the best life. Savulescu insists that as tests for non-disease genes become available, parents have emerging moral obligations to use them in making decisions about reproduction. This is a technological imperative reminiscent of Buchanan *et al.*'s image of the "colonization" of justice (2000, 82–84).

Savulescu does claim that those who want a child with diminished well-being, and have good reason for this desire, can choose to have such a child from his perspective (2001b, 424–425). Consider his published opinion in the case of Sharon Duchesneau and Candy McCullough, a deaf lesbian couple who used a deaf sperm donor they selected specifically to ensure that the child they created would be deaf. In that case, he claimed that people should be free to do what they want unless it harms others. Since the child Duchesneau and McCullough created would not otherwise exist, the child cannot be said to be harmed by its own creation (cf. Parfit 1984). That means that Duchesneau and McCullough should, Savulescu argues, be free to have a deaf child (Savulescu 2002). Since Savulescu specifies that his sense of "moral" with regard to procreative beneficence specifies what we have good reason to do when good reasons to do otherwise are absent, he seems to believe Duchesneau and McCullough had sufficient reason to justify their choice.[1] Despite this explicit support, the calculus of procreative beneficence devised by Savulescu still requires that the existence of persons with disabilities be explained and justified.

Savulescu clarifies that his support of liberty in these cases "does not imply that there are no normative principles to guide these choices" (2001b, 425). In light of this, despite the fact that Savulescu claims advocates for reproductive liberty in the case of Duchesneau and McCullough, he argues that medical professionals leading parents through screening practices and selection procedures should try to persuade them to follow the dictates of procreative beneficence (2001b, 425). While individuals must personally balance their own procreative liberty against the duty of procreative beneficence, medical professionals should advocate for selection on the basis of information drawn from any available genetic testing and technology (425; cf. Savulescu 2002). The linkage between medical professionals and genetic selection advocacy generates status for genetic selection as a science and translates Savulescu's assessment of what counts as the best life into a kind of scientific objectivity. Like Fisher and Fisk, the scientists of the Life Extension Institute at the turn of the century, Savulescu believes his notions of wanted and unwanted traits are undeniable and matters of biology. Savulescu endorses ableist prejudice as justifiable when he writes that he does not believe that those who already live with disabilities are less valuable; he just wants to reduce the number of children born with disabilities. He also suggests that "savings from selection against embryos/fetuses with genetic abnormalities to improving well-being of existing people with disabilities" (2001b, 423). This, like other transhumanist visions, takes for granted the desirability of a future without disability (cf. Kafer 2011).

Savulescu does admit that procreative beneficence allows common prejudices to come into play in reproductive decision-making. But, his response to the problem is unsatisfactory. He argues that if society favors men, then parents have good moral reason to select embryos based on their sex (male) (2001b, 423). But, he does not think that these decisions impact equality or justice issues, because before any impact is felt on the level of the population, emergent factors (i.e. gender disparity) would change the direction of moral obligation (*ibid.*). He argues that in a society which has produced too many males, but still relies on traditional sexual reproduction, a female child becomes the favored outcome of a pregnancy under the dictates of procreative beneficence. Yet, this feels like a red herring, because Savulescu seems to simultaneously advocate against traditional reproduction.

Persons with disabilities, women, people of color, and others who face oppression, have important reasons to be suspicious of Savulescu's procreative beneficence. It is clear people of color experience significantly worse societal reception and conditions than those positioned as white, so Savulescu appears forced to argue that one should select for biological "whiteness" (against a "raced" fetus). Despite his treatment of the "deaf lesbians" case, he does not deal adequately with ableism and sexism. Savulescu's focus on eliminating undesirable traits biologically obscures the ways in which disability involves a lack of fit to or lack of responsiveness in a particular social world, which is malleable, or is socially constructed by way of stigma. Marking disability is a labeling and naming process; labels in turn come to refer to the whole person in a disparaging way: "the amputee" or the Down's baby—a "defect" becomes a "defective" (cf. Zola 1993, 169). Marking procedures are a major element of the social construction of disability identity, and are stigmatizing practices.

Finally, Savulescu does not bring into view the women who would be receiving the in vitro fertilization (IVF) treatments necessary to enact the principle of procreative beneficence (he typically refers to "reproducers" rather than "women"). Noting this concern, bioethicist Christine Overall argues that procreative beneficence is a burden for women, not men because procreative beneficence requires "every potential mother" to use IVF (Overall 2012, 125). But, IVF involves major surgeries and so procreative beneficence is in actuality a high-risk medical experiment for both the mother and the child. Risks to the fetus stem from the likelihood of multiples brought by the IVF procedure, and so when IVF is combined with preimplantation diagnosis, an improved life for a potential child cannot be guaranteed. To reiterate: a procedure undertaken in the name of avoiding future risk to the fetus creates immediate risk. These issues are all beside the point, however, for the majority of women globally; we should not forget that IVF is extremely cost-prohibitive (125–127). On a basic level, IVF is incredibly resource-heavy, and prenatal genetic diagnosis involves deep freezers, complex lab equipment, and a team of doctors. Procreative beneficence is meant to be an ethical principle—on Savulescu's view, the morally correct way to reproduce—but it fails with regard to bettering the lives of precisely those whose participation it requires (Overall 2012, 127).

THE DISABILITY CRITIQUE OF NEGATIVE GENETIC SELECTION

Scholar Adrienne Asch critiques the practice of negative genetic selection by claiming that selecting against traits deemed characteristic of already-existing persons[2] with disabilities is deeply stigmatizing and sends a hurtful message to those in the disability community (2003). On Asch's view, then, procreative beneficence would be immoral, and Savulescu's commitment to both valuing already-existing persons with disabilities and refusing to create new persons with disabilities falls apart. In what follows, I describe Asch's view and extend it into a critique of procreative beneficence. I also deepen it by reference to genetic determinism and stigma. The disability critique I discuss here should in no sense be taken as somehow representative of a monolithic "disabled voice" or "disability community." The *disability critique* is the term for a specific argument promoted by Asch (Asch 1989, 2000, 2003; Asch and Wasserman 2005).

In her disability critique, Asch claims that negative genetic selection is regularly undertaken by individuals based on misinformation ultimately related to ableism, is unduly swayed by the medical model of disability, and expresses a hurtful message to persons already-existing with targeted disability traits—namely, that these lives are not worth living. For supporters of the critique, "prenatal genetic testing followed by selective abortion is morally problematic, and . . . driven by misinformation" (Parens and Asch 2000, 13). Asch further suggests that if disability is seen to detract from "what most people seek in child rearing," which she specifies as a process "to give ourselves a new being who starts out with the best we can give, and who will enrich us, gladden others, contribute to the world, and make us proud," then this is a result of misinformation (13, quoting Asch 1989, 86). So, the misinformation that Asch has in mind is connected to evaluations about the character of the child that might be created and, additionally, the way in which rearing that child would be different or unique from rearing any child (see also Kittay 2010c).

The misinformation identified by the disability critique can take a number of different forms, but is shaped by both disregard for the value of the lives of persons with disabilities and biased quality of life judgments. Asch writes:

> Clinicians and bioethicists often discount data indicating that people with disabilities and their families do not view their lives in solely or even predominantly negative terms; instead, they may insist that such data reflect a denial of reality or an exceptional ability to cope with problems. (Parens and Asch 2000, 6; see also Riis *et al.* 2005; Goering 2008)

Relatedly, researchers in the social sciences have investigated the operation of "impact bias," that is, "a tendency to overestimate the influence that events will have on one's QOL [quality of life]" (Smith *et al.* 2008, 653). They found that in the case of kidney transplants, those who undergo the surgery overestimate the impact that the surgery will have on their quality of life (2008). In fact, they found that patients succumb to the same "spreading effect" I discussed in Chapter 2, in other words, "people may over generalize the improvement that would occur in health status to other areas. Indeed, we found that some of the most optimistic predictions for improvements were in areas that did not change at all after transplant, such as employment and travel" (657). The researchers go on to suggest that it would be interesting to see how this "spreading effect" impacts quality of life prediction with regard to perceived negative events, like disability—they wonder, will individuals "believe that disability will negatively affect areas of life that will actually be relatively unaffected?" (Smith *et al.* 2008, 658). This certainly appears to be the case in bioethics literature.

One "mistaken assumption" Asch discusses at length is the assumption that if having a capacity is good, then lacking it is inherently bad. Asch argues that one can concede a capacity is valuable without conceding that to live without it is bad, or lacking in value. Equivocation between these two beliefs makes the "quality of life" of those with disabilities seem unduly low or perhaps non-existent. This problem is linked to "overly narrow" descriptions of what counts as a good life (2003, 318). We can see this narrowness in Savulescu's argumentation; he zeros in on cognitive capacity as a key factor which can ensure a valuable life (e.g. Savulescu 2001b). The importance of cognitive capacity in Savulescu's argument finds support elsewhere in bioethics literature; for example, Buchanan *et al.* argue that cognitive capacity is "all-purpose" and so does not define a particular life of value, but is rather necessary to all (2000, 49). Transhumanist arguments for intellectual enhancement define cognitive ability as necessarily valuable and implicitly claim that greater cognitive capacity is always better. This means higher IQ is of vital importance (Savulescu 2001b, 414). This assumption necessarily devalues the lives of those with intellectual disabilities.

Asch identifies two other factors which perpetuate misinformation. First, discriminatory attitudes toward persons with disabilities are driven by the medical model of disability (2003, 318–19). Insofar as negative genetic selection is explicitly encouraged by medical professionals as a way of avoiding a life of hardship, Asch argues a medical model is likely being employed, which exaggerates the extent to which negative experiences often undergone by persons with disabilities are due inherently to their physical traits. Recall that the medical model of disability, on its strongest version, orients all limitation due to disability in biological facts; discomforts and lack of freedoms and limited capabilities are all, on this model, due solely to disability's character as a medical or health problem (Brownlee and Cureton 2009, 75–76; Saxton 2000, 149). Rejecting this emphasis, as proponents of disability rights usually do, can take the form of assuming a largely social model of disability or simply rejecting the medical model. Contrary to the medical model, the social model argues that difficulties or differences in quality of life experienced by persons with disabilities are due to a lack of social accommodation rather than inherent individual or biological qualities (Abberley 1987). Recall that disability, on this view, most closely refers to a set of social circumstances that are discriminatory rather than a trait or traits of an individual or the individual herself (Brownlee and Cureton 2009, 21). This does not mean that the traits in question must be seen as neutral; this shift in emphasis can still consider certain traits limiting in connection with some activities and at the same time maintain that available alternative modes of activity can translate into a high quality of life (Parens and Asch 2000, 25–26). The disability critique suggests, then, that a disability trait *need not* have the "tragic" impact it is regularly believed to have as viewed through the medical model, if social acceptance and accommodations are available.

Second, negative genetic selection "place[s] unwarranted emphasis on the size of one's opportunity range rather than the possibility for meaningful choice and rewarding outcomes within that range" (Asch 2003, 318). Recall here Bostrom's image of concentric circles, the larger of which represents the opportunity range of posthumans, while the smaller represents that of humans. Using the language of the species-typical, Asch points out that variation from this norm does not mean that "meaningful choice and rewarding outcomes" are lost. In fact, "virtually everyone with a disability can participate in many everyday activities, experience relationships, discover the world beyond themselves, and contribute to familial, social, political, and economic life" (320). An over-emphasis on opportunity range ensconces "meaningful choice and rewarding outcomes" as inherent to the life of an individual who enjoys a body considered more species-typical, or a specific kind of genotype. This emphasis *over-valuates* the opportunity range of the (socially) abled body, while simultaneously *denying* the opportunity range of the (socially) disabled body.

Any individual may face hospital stays, obstacles, chronic illness, disease, or permanent limitation. Yet, society is only responsive to some needs, not all, and creates circumstances in which some persons are more accepted and cared for than others. Opportunity ranges can enforce a misleading binary between the disabled and the abled and, in the context of prenatal testing, encourage predictions impossible to make. Quality of life is utterly dependent upon social circumstances, so prenatal testing cannot predict it. And notice again that the selection and enhancement rhetoric emphasizes choice—what is opportunity range but a field of proliferating choices?[3]

The disability critique also critically assesses synecdoche, the identification of one trait with the whole, that is, the whole fetus or the entirety of the prospects of the future child (Parens and Asch 2000, 14 and 27–28; Asch and Wasserman 2005). Asch sees synecdoche as yet another conceptual mistake which ties the value of an entire fetus or future child to the presence of a trait that has been socially identified as problematic or unwelcome. The rejection of a fetus, then, is by way of synecdoche predicated on the presence of one trait. Through the lens of synecdoche, Savulescu's procreative beneficence assumes that the presence of one trait thought to impact quality of life is enough to make an embryo undesirable. Rich possibilities regarding potential persons are obscured. These embryos are marked by stigma; recall Coleman Brown's formulation of stigma as "the attribute that colors the perception of the entire person" (2010, 184).

On my view, we should make a distinction between preventing harm for a particular child and preventing a particular child in order to avoid the existence of a disability. To put it yet another way, there is a distinction between preventing harm (through the use of folic acid, for example) on behalf of a child or a potential child, and preventing a potential child because of an unwanted trait (cf. Parens and Asch 2000, 16). Savulescu conflates the distinction I am trying to make when he writes: "It is important to distinguish between disability and persons with disability. Selection reduces the former, but is silent on the value of the latter" (2001b, 423). The difference is one of emphasis, which hearkens back to the concept of synecdoche. Preventing a potential child because of an unwanted trait can point to an undue belief in the influence of that trait, which in turn may be inflated by undercurrents of genetic determinism. It is also a thoroughly biopolitical practice, one which presumes what types of lives are worth living and fixates on preventing specific bodies rather than adjusting social institutions.

Genetic determinism, again, is the latest in a string of biological reductions haunting the last century of enhancement thinking. Genetic determinism assumes that wide swaths of behavior and social phenomena can be explained solely through biological factors. The synecdoche connected with prenatal testing insists that future quality of life can be measured, at least in the present time, through the presence or absence of certain genetic traits, markers or indicators. Savulescu claims that quality of life can be predicted reliably by reference to genetic data, and these predictions should be actionable. This is part of a strategy of actuarial thinking in reproductive technology that links with Savulescu's discursive emphasis on choice; for him, morality requires that parents "choose" high quality of life for future children; this clearly over-emphasizes the importance of genetic factors. It showcases a bias toward genetic impact factors over those of environment and society.

To put these issues a slightly different way: genetic determinism positions genetic cause as ruling over individual outcome. Synecdoche, likewise, positions a "disability" trait as absolute or autonomous limitation upon individual quality of life. Synecdoche identifies one trait of the fetus as of utmost importance. It makes this partial information about genotype appear to enable the choice for or against a particular kind of a child, seen primarily through the lens of genetic traits. Using only the lens of genetic traits belies the known influences of environment, the complicated relationship between genotype and phenotype, and the fallibility of genetic predictors (Gupta 2012; Kolata 2012). Genetic selection, seen as the choice of outcomes in quality of life rather than intervention upon mere traits, would provide a potential parent with a child who is chosen as opposed to one that is the product of chance.

The other elements of misinformation I drew out from Asch's work, above, are also linked to biological reductionism. First, the notion that lack is always negative or that the size of one's predicted opportunity range is of primary importance relies on the idea that *biology is destiny*—certain physical facts about one's body will always determine the type of life one leads. This resonates with the history of enhancement I drew in the previous chapter.

Second, the medical model attributes primary importance to the physical facts of one's body, while disregarding the extent to which accessibility, stigma and bias in the social world can contribute to, or work against, one's quality of life.

A selected genotype, taken as a guarantor of a better child (one closer to society's vision), positions genetic factors as if they uniquely determine phenotype, opportunity range, and quality of life. Taken as a kind of guarantee—the "selection" of a child or a life—a genotype selected for or against appears to stave off unpredictability and chance. In a recent case in the state of Oregon, parents launched a multi-million-dollar lawsuit against a hospital for failing to detect Down syndrome in their then 4-year-old daughter. The parents claim that they were "assured" that the results of tests for the condition were negative (Heasley 2012). If it were not for the notion of a guarantee when testing *does not* uncover a trait that parents wish to avoid, such suits would not be successful in court (cf. Shiffrin 1999). Parents may feel that through genetic selection they are choosing a life of unbounded possibility as opposed to known or absolute limitation. But, this is an illusion—selecting against specific traits does not guarantee future happiness or an untroubled life.

Rosemarie Garland-Thomson refers to the opposite of the abnormal as the *normate*, an empty point of reference that no one embodies. Again, linking this insight to genetic determinism can deepen this discussion. "Normal" genotypes also function as empty points of reference; there is no person with a genotypic "blueprint for normal phenotype" (Scully 2008, 6). Negative genetic selection, as a cultural practice today, reinforces the normate in terms of genotype and connects this construct with individual happiness or quality of life. "Canonical genotypes" are conceptual constructs built by social and cultural values, and deviance is filled out by way of what society refuses to tolerate. The basis for "normality" is imaginative—it connects biological causes to what are considered to be desirable outcomes, which in turn represent desirable characteristics. These desirable characteristics always have reference to the social world and its delineation between normal and abnormal, acceptable and stigmatized. Like the "normate" (the "unblushing," abled, heterosexual, educated male who is Christian, plays sports—the list goes on, Garland-Thomson 1996, 9)—the canonical genotype is empty. No one person is owner of the "canonical genotype"—variation is constant (Scheer and Groce 1998).

There is no reason to believe that widespread use of enhancements, even genetic selection, would create an orderly Gattacan world of unbounded successes, happiness, and pure opportunity. Hope that it might, expressed by enhancement proponents, expresses at least genetic bias if not full-blown support for genetic determinism. Lurking in the background is the idea that a selected genotype produces a predictable set of results and is susceptible to manipulation through pure choice and no chance (Oliver 2010). Hope that genetic intervention can at least guarantee lives of fewer obstacles, burdens, or less suffering, also expresses genetic bias. Savulescu is working from genetic bias when he advocates selection for traits connected to enhanced cognition, no matter how weak the link between genotype and phenotype, or how "accurate" the tests for intelligence (2001, 414). Genetic interventions are costly and time-consuming, both for individuals and for societies that invest in their use. If, for Savulescu, they are important enough to advocate for and invest in even when the linkage between genes and quality of life is weak, as he argues, he positions these interventions among many other social and political investment strategies as primarily important (2001b). Perhaps, then, these strategies are useful as a result of the bodies they reject, not the bodies they create.

On a final line of argumentation generally referred to as the *expressivist view*, advocates of the disability critique contend that prenatal testing and genetic selection, as attitude and practice, send a hurtful message to already-existing persons with the traits in question (Saxton 2000, 148; Asch 2000b, 236). Asch clarifies: "As with discrimination more generally, with prenatal diagnosis, a single trait stands in for the whole, the trait obliterates the whole. With both discrimination and prenatal diagnosis, nobody finds out about the rest. *The tests send the message that there's no need to find out about the rest*" (Parens and Asch 2000, 13; emphasis mine). This message tells already-existing persons that their lives are not worth living. Ultimately, Asch suggests that "trying to screen for and prevent the birth" of those with certain traits "disparage[s] the lives of existing and future disabled people" who share these traits (Parens and Asch 2000, 13). It also misconstrues their lives. Synecdoche upholds this message by prioritizing single traits over future wholes. Asch and David Wasserman suggest that synecdoche is a moral "failing" (notice that they do not mean the act of negative genetic selection itself, although they might mean a parental ethic or attitude behind an act) (2005, 173).

Asch and Wasserman, along with others who articulate or adhere to the disability critique, recognize that not all instances of selective abortion must be interpreted as ableist or motivated by stereotyping and stigma. Asch and Parens write: "Parents may examine themselves and conclude that they are not choosing against a child's specific traits; they may be making an honest and informed acceptance of their own character and goals" (Parens and Asch 2000, 22; cf. Asch and Wasserman 2005). Individual women may make an assessment of their circumstances in light of the results of prenatal testing and determine that they do not have the resources, social support or otherwise have access to the tools necessary to raise a particular child. This should not be read as a failure of an individual woman, as some versions of the disability critique might suggest. Instead it should be a jumping-off point for a searching investigation of what forms of life society welcomes and a motivation to begin working politically to make the distribution of medical care, housing, and other social goods more just and equitable—which might in turn transform the assessment parents make tools available to raise particular children. While the disability critique is not usually used to inspire this conversation, it can and should be. We can foster better lives for our children by choosing to engage in social transformation.

REPRODUCTIVE LIBERTY AND JUSTICE

It is important to return, however, to the conflict I discussed at the outset of this chapter. Some object to the disability critique, and may object to my extension of it, because it appears to restrict reproductive choice (Brock 2009; Nelson 2011; and Savulescu 2001b). If it is ethically permissible to terminate a pregnancy, it is permissible to terminate any pregnancy for any reason (Brock 2009, 258; Steinbock 2000). Savulescu posits that claims like the disability critique require parents unwilling to raise disabled children to create and support such children (2001b, 423). He assumes that proponents of the *disability discrimination claim* (as he calls it) support a ban on genetic selection procedures and selective abortion in response to the presence of certain traits (*ibid.*). Like Savulescu, Jamie Nelson views the disability critique as inimical to reproductive liberty and rejects the idea that any amount of stigma suffered by existing persons could be sufficient reason to force an unwanted pregnancy (2010). Daniel Brock has argued that even if one assumes the expressivist view is correct to claim that negative genetic selection involves a hurtful message sent to already-existing persons, the disability critique poses a threat to reproductive liberty (2009, 258). Steinbock argues that the decision to selectively abort on the basis of a disability trait is acceptable for the same reason any abortion is acceptable: so the woman is not forced to take on unwanted burdens (2000, 119).

But, disability advocates interested in promoting a version of the disability critique need not subscribe to a view that precludes reproductive liberty in individual cases (i.e., advocating forced pregnancies) to voice concern regarding the marginalization, stigmatization, and prejudicial attitudes developed and expressed through the social practice of genetic selection on the basis of disability traits (Parens and Asch 2000, 12). To assume otherwise is to reduce the disability critique to a straw man. In fact, Asch holds that potential parent(s) should be the primary decision-makers regarding their reproductive liberty (Parens and Asch 2000, 22; cf. Asch 2003, 317 n. 6 and 332–34). She writes: "I, and nearly all others sharing a disability rights critique of prenatal testing, maintain an ardent pro-choice stance and assert that women should be free to make any decision they wish about maintaining a pregnancy or having an abortion" (2003, 317 n. 6). As bioethicist Erik Parens and Asch articulate the critique:

> The disability community arguments are not intended to justify wholesale restrictions on prenatal testing for genetic disability. Rather, they are intended to make prospective parents pause and think about what they are doing and to challenge professionals to help parents better examine their decisions. They [should] help make our decisions *thoughtful and informed, not thoughtless and automatic.* (2000, 28–29, emphasis mine)

The best outcome, from the standpoint of the disability critique, is that potential parents, having resolved to have children, reflect carefully on what testing can reveal about their future child.

Against Savulescu, reflection should not be burdened by undue coercion from medical professionals, which can devolve into a shaming process and contribute to systemic marginalization and prejudice. I am thinking specifically of situations like one in which a genetic counselor reportedly asked an expectant mother, "What are you going to say to people when they ask you how you could bring a child like this into the world?" (Parens and Asch 2000, 7). Or, in another example, an obstetrician remarked to a woman that "the quickest, cheapest way to solve this problem is to terminate the pregnancy" (reported in Piepmeier 2013). Instead, medical professionals should encourage reflection and take care not to overstate the predictive power of genetic testing.

Differences presented by and the necessity for social accommodations for particular traits should not be downplayed. It is, however, of utmost importance to neither overstate the importance of genetic factors among others in connection with quality of life, nor accept and amplify the effects of prejudice and stigma against persons with disabilities, by treating these effects as inherent to certain traits without reference to the social institutions and circumstances which actually create them. The lack of social accommodations for particular traits is not a natural circumstance and can be transformed.

Reproductive liberty is dependent upon reliable information from medical professionals and a non-coercive setting in which to make reproductive decisions. Bias toward genetic definitions of opportunity range or the undue belief in genetic determinism actually thwart these conditions. Both can complicate the transmission of good information, foster misinformation, and put undue pressure on potential parents. Importantly, there is no reliable medical information about quality of life. No matter how good or predictive prenatal testing becomes, no matter how perfect the transmission of information between a medical professional and a woman, predictions like this are inaccessible. Again, this is because the richness of one's life, the access one enjoys to others and to the world, is dependent upon social and political responsiveness, just conditions, and the acceptance of diverse embodiment.

Further, I see the push to engage in negative genetic selection and prenatal testing practices as continuous with the biopolitical rhetoric around healthy choices that restrict pregnant women. Healthy food choices made by women who are pregnant are considered one guarantor of a healthy (read: abled) fetus, and dietary restrictions discipline a woman's diet with precision. In fact, women's consumption of food and drink during pregnancy is subject to evolving, and at times, bizarre and punishing, proscriptions. For instance, pregnant women have been refused rice, instructed not to drink tap water, soft cheeses and cured meats, and warned about risks to the fetus if women eat seafood while pregnant (Sutton, Douglas and McClellan 2011 and Meyer-Rochow 2009; Murphy *et al.* 2011, 812–814). Despite lack of evidence with regard to risk, women are told to abstain from alcohol and caffeine. When refusing to follow these guidelines, women must swallow stigma and guilt (Murphy *et al.* 2011, 812). Social scientists have suggested that both hostile and benevolent sexism is to blame (813). It is difficult to see prenatal testing as part of women's access to reproductive liberty when it perpetuates ableism and is continuous with sexist and intrusive monitoring of women's choices. Think again of news personality Bree Walker Lampley who was criticized as irresponsible after she stated her intention to continue a pregnancy when the resulting child would have ectrodactyly (Parens and Asch 2000, 8). In the transhumanist version of reproduction choice, women are immoral and irresponsible if they make the "wrong" choice. The woman is positioned as uniquely able to affect the character, nature, phenotype, or ability of the fetus, and so her every behavior during the time of pregnancy is open to scrutiny and regulation. The mother is thought to provide both the form (genes) and content (environment) of her future child. Sexism and ableism are here intertwined.

On my view, the appropriate target of a critique of negative genetic selection is not women who choose to abort but discourse in medical and scientific realms which exacerbates the influence of genetic determinism or takes recourse to an unmitigated medical mode of disability. Effective critique would counter the lack of reflection upon synecdoche in social and institutional encouragement to select. This reorientation reflects bioethicist Christine Overall's desire to question practices rather than preferences (1987). Finally, the disability critique should be used to help us recognize the need to pair critique of these issues with activism aimed toward social and political changes in medical care, insurance, public policy, transportation, accommodation, and schools. We need to create a more just system to alleviate marginalization of and discrimination against persons with disabilities. So many social situations effectively "hide" persons with disabilities from view—I think of institutions like sheltered workshops, relegation to nursing homes, and extreme lack of public transportation.

Here again, a model of disability, like the cultural model, which can attend to social constructions of disability and stigmas against persons with disabilities is a requirement. Unfair stereotyping of disability occurs when one naturalizes or materializes disability—that is, conflates social constructions regarding persons and groups, and stigmas connected with these, with facts about the body. I take synecdoche to be the most significant insight of the original disability critique; synecdoche naturalizes and stigmatizes by focusing merely on rejected traits themselves, as materializations of disability, and so prioritizes isolated traits over social circumstances as primarily important. Synecdoche hides what is in plain sight from view.

Bioethicist Jamie Nelson rejects the idea that selective termination can be read as a hurtful message to existing persons. She writes:

> people's motivations and reasons, their understandings and aims, are so various as to preclude our being able to say "this behavior can only be understood as sending a resentment-worthy message." Abortions after genetic screenings are not sentences, nor are they even symbols—and even if they were, of course, what people mean in using sentences, or in running flags up poles, is various and contestable. (2011, 66)

Nelson goes on to argue that motivations for terminating a fetus with a disability trait "will typically be less hateful" than those motivations that proponents of the disability critique might argue are behind genetic selection (67). Yet, as I have argued so far, I think that the focus of the disability critique is better rested upon the aggregate social impact of negative genetic selection than upon women or individuals making decisions. I concede that it would be unfair and very likely incorrect to insist on arguing that particular individuals are driven by hateful motivations when they decide to terminate particular pregnancies. Instead, it seems most helpful and best to argue, especially in the context of transhumanist utopias, that the social practice of genetic selection and the particular urgings of the medical community have the effect of large-scale commentary on which lives are worth living and which bodies society wishes to produce. While "abortions after genetic screenings are not sentences," genetic counselors and medical professionals speak sentences, internet resources post sentences ("running flags up poles"), and in most cases these and other sentences are both uniformly ableist and have tangible effects on individual decision-making (66).

Individual women cannot be morally expected, at the moment they are faced with the results of prenatal testing, to alone recognize and weed out the impact of the unfair and false binary between abled and disabled with regard to life opportunities, as well as the influence of genetic determinism. The key drawback of past promotion of the disability critique is the focus in some articulations of the critique on messages sent by individual women's decision-making rather than institutions as a whole (cf. Asch and Gellner 1996, 339; Hershey 1994, 30 as quoted in Nelson 2007, 478). My expansion of the critique to include the notion of genetic determinism as a common fallacy with an impact on medical discourse and the provision of care is meant to adjust this claim beyond individual reproducers and the decisions they may make. Decisions made by individual parents are currently unduly influenced by unsupported belief in the idea that genetic profiles taken before birth have measurable and certain impact on future quality of life as well as ableism in an unresponsive society.

Philosopher Licia Carlson notes that other bioethicists, including Allan Buchanan and Laura Purdy, argue that the disability critique's expressivist view—the idea that selection against certain traits sends a harmful message—fails because of the "conceptual separation between traits and persons" (207). But, she argues, these critics have not done enough when they merely assert this separation, "given the complex relationship between disabling conditions and self-identity described by persons with disabilities" (207). Further, she argues, "this distinction between qualities and persons cannot be made at the prenatal level" (207). She clarifies: "the separation between qualities and persons is impossible when the only means of eliminating the trait is abortion" (207). According to Carlson:

> The etiologic paradox of this new screening technology is that the genotype or chromosomal anomaly is visible prenatally, yet its phenotypic manifestation remains invisible until the child is born or years later (depending on the condition). I maintain that this indeterminacy creates the possibility of what I call prenatal prototypes: cases which are applied prenatally but are taken as representative of an entire class of future persons. (208)

For Carlson, then, genetic profiles taken of an embryo or fetus in screening procedures encourage the development of "prenatal prototypes" (2002, 207–209).

Relatedly, screening methods and fetal diagnostics are a naming process, by which a fetus is connected to an already-existing group. A medical professional may explain to a potential parent that their baby will have Down syndrome, for example, which will call forward the figures of already-existing persons as a set of references. Marsha Saxton suggests that "when we refer to the fetus as a 'disabled fetus' . . . the fetus is named as a member of our [disability] community" (2000, 159). If this calling forward were literal, involving meeting and getting to know actual members of the disability community, perhaps progress could be made. The calling forward, however, is merely symbolic; medical professionals name by way of diagnosis, which involves medicalizing the predicted condition of the potential person.[4] Saxton, referring to the work of Hershey, notes that "medical language reinforces negativity." For Hershey, "terms like 'fetal deformity' and 'defective fetus' are deeply stigmatizing, carrying connotations of inadequacy and shame" (as quoted and discussed in Saxton 2000, 149). Medical practice, she contends, also tends to unfairly view the disabled as *permanent patients* who are "subject to the definitions and control of the medical profession" (*ibid.*, cf. Scheer and Groce 1998, 34). Again, critique of the medical model is helpful. Persons with disabilities are patients sometimes, as are persons who are abled. Viewing the disabled as permanent patients ignores universal vulnerability and contributes to a fundamental binary between the abled and disabled. Most importantly, it is marginalizing and inaccurate.

Angela Davis and other feminists of color concerned about the rhetoric of choice in abortion politics raise an important distinction between reproductive liberty and reproductive justice, which calls into question precisely the issue at hand: the failure to extend questions about reproductive choices beyond the sphere of individual liberty (Davis 1981; see also Smith 2005). For Davis, "the failure of the abortion rights campaign to conduct a historical self-evaluation led to a dangerously superficial appraisal of Black people's suspicious attitudes toward birth control in general. Granted, when some Black people unhesitatingly equated birth control with genocide, it did appear to be an exaggerated—even paranoiac—reaction" (1981, 203). But Davis goes on to claim that "white abortion rights activists" missed available "clues about the history of the birth control movement" in the strong reactions of the black community (1981, 203–204). Historically, the birth control movement advocated racist, involuntary sterilization; this advocacy extended to Margaret Sanger, the engine of the movement in the 1900s, and Theodore Roosevelt, U.S. president at the turn of the century (204, 209, and 210). For Davis—writing in the 1980s—until involuntary sterilization and racism were substantially addressed and rejected in the abortion rights movement, reproductive liberty was non-existent for many women. She argued: "if ever women would enjoy the right to plan their pregnancies, legal and easily accessible birth control measures and abortions would have to be complemented by an end to sterilization abuse" (204).

The sterilization abuse to which Davis refers was sanctioned and enjoyed broad support both within and beyond the birth control movement in recent history. Involuntary sterilization laws were in effect in many states in the 1930s; "By 1932 . . . at least twenty-six states had passed compulsory sterilization laws and . . . thousands of 'unfit' persons had already been surgically prevented from reproducing" (1981, 214; cf. Snyder and Mitchell 2006, 98). Margaret Sanger affirmed this state of affairs when she announced that the sterilization was right for: "Morons, mental defectives, epileptics, illiterates, paupers, unemployables, criminals, prostitutes and dope fiends" (as quoted in Davis 1981, 214). Davis adds that Sanger believed that if sterilization were refused, these persons "should be able to choose a lifelong segregated existence in labor camps" (*ibid.*).

Sterilization abuse has an analog in the history of slavery; for black women under slave conditions, abortion was not a solution, but a way to ensure that no children of their own would be brought into slavery, physical abuse, and sexual abuse (1981, 204). For them, "abortions and infanticides were acts of desperation, motivated not by the biological birth process but by the oppressive conditions of slavery. Most of these women, no doubt, would have expressed their deepest resentment had someone hailed their abortions as a stepping stone toward freedom" (205). For Davis, in order to succeed and unite women, the abortion rights movement needed to critically examine the historical conditions of forced abortions and sterilizations and acknowledge the impact of these conditions on attitudes among people of color toward abortion rights. Including a condemnation of sterilization abuse would have saved the movement in the 1970s, Davis argues (1981, 215).

Davis introduces a distinction between birth control and population control; the latter was an outgrowth of eugenic thinking and defeated the "progressive potential" of the birth control movement, which should have "[advocated] for people of color . . . the individual right to birth control" but instead refused to address the historical complexities that made people of color the intended victims of eugenic birth control (1981, 215).

Persons with disabilities, like people of color, are historically the victims of compulsory sterilization laws in the United States and elsewhere around the world (Snyder and Mitchell 2006, 30, 86, 91, 127, and 186). By the year 1963, it is estimated that 63,000 individuals considered disabled had been "forcibly sterilized" in state institutions (86). Additionally, those with disabilities have fallen victim (and still fall victim) to a system of marginalizing institutionalization in sheltered workshops, nursing homes, and group homes that packs a triple threat of segregation, oppression, and underpaid labor (Diament 2012a, 2012b). The sexuality of these individuals is today still controlled as part of their isolation in nursing homes and institutions. Snyder and Mitchell comment that, starting in the late 1890s through the turn of the century,

> Institutional practices explicitly sought to extract defective citizens from participation in the social mainstream. In this regard, institutions for the feebleminded . . . in conjunction with the passage of marriage and state sterilization laws, eugenics institutions participated in erasing disabled citizens from public view with the full sanction of state and federal governments. (2006, 91)

The institutional practices in question also involved a type of incarceration which made "public intimacy" impossible, and "posed as safe, humane places for the 'treatment' of disabilities while operating essentially as research warehouses" (2006, 91). The continued history of forced and permanent institutionalization of persons with disabilities, working along with the compulsory sterilization laws that were common in the first half of the twentieth century, parallel the experience of people of color with sterilization and slavery. Both additionally experienced, and in the case of persons with disabilities, still experience restrictions on marriage as a result of these institutions and oppressive laws (cf. Snyder and Mitchell 2006, 127; see also the story of the couple Paul Forziano and Hava Samuels, who sued the federal government to live together after being refused that right by their separate group homes, in Heasley 2013).

The distinction between birth control and population control is very helpful in the case of disability rights; some disability rights activists and scholars now claim, just as people of color claimed in the 1970s, that what some view as the simple exercise of reproductive rights (genetic selection) is akin to genocide (e.g. Marcia Bristo as quoted in Montgomery 1999). Just like in the former case, a full account of reproductive *justice* requires awareness and rejection of injustice, historical and current, perpetrated against persons with disabilities. A further parallel between the two: one justification for the racist application of what Davis refers to as "mass 'birth control'" (1981, 204) was the supposed hyper-fertility and simultaneous poverty of people of color (209–210, 213–214). Similarly, those with assumed cognitive disability were long considered more fertile—and thus in need of containment—than others: "the feebleminded woman who marries is twice as prolific as the normal woman" (1912 document, as quoted in Snyder and Mitchell 2006, 186). In personal correspondence, Sanger admitted that an ultimate goal of the birth control movement was to "exterminate the Negro population" (as quoted in Davis 19821, 125).

To draw my comparison to a close, I note Sharon Snyder and David Mitchell's interpretation of the intent of marriage restriction, sterilization and segregation in the case of persons with disabilities. They write: "the legacy of eugenics was sweeping, systematic, and violently pathologizing because it founded its interventions on the mistaken faith in the ability to eradicate what is believed to be undesirable degrees of physical and cognitive differences from the biological record" (2006, 86). The push for genetic selection is based on the same mistaken faith, and the faith involved relies on genetic determinism for its strength. Human enhancement through genetic selection is bent on the eradication of difference. On my view, any critique of or intervention upon *only* individuals who plan to reproduce will be insufficient and also highly problematic. Instead, powerful and effective critiques must be institutional. They must focus on the discourse and rhetoric that poses genetic selection as a *choice* for better future humans, framing it within reproductive liberty. This is parallel to the framing of involuntary sterilization within the abortion rights movement of the previous century. We must also focus on making our world more accessible to and accepting of diverse forms of embodiment.

The disability critique can expose pervasive injustices facing those in the disability community on the basis of belief in genetic determinism and the pressure on potential parents to test for and select for, or selectively abort in response to, disability traits. As disability activist Laura Hershey writes, "We struggle for integration, access, and support services, yet our existence remains an unresolved question. Under the circumstances, we cannot expect society to guarantee and fund our full citizenship" (as quoted in Saxton 2000, 153–4). Social support of and investment in research regarding testing and selecting procedures for disability traits seems to preclude or at least complicate investment in accessible social spaces and needed services for existing persons with disabilities (cf. Asch 2003).

TRANSHUMANISM AND DISABILITY RIGHTS

Given my discussion in this book so far, it is hard to imagine transhumanists as allies in disability rights projects. But, some claim the potential for such an alliance. *Fixed: The Science/Fiction of Human Enhancement*, a recent documentary by independent filmmaker Regan Brashear depicts this potential alliance between transhumanists and disabled persons (2013). Transhumanists have claimed persons with disabilities as part of their movement and have described themselves as allies in the fight for disability rights (Dvorsky 2003; *Fixed* 2013; Hughes 2009; Wasserman 2012). Simultaneously, some disabled individuals, like Gregor Wolbring, promote radical enhancement as a path toward fighting disability oppression, or, perhaps, toward making oppression irrelevant through the dissolution of plausible distinctions between abled and disabled (Wolbring 2009; cf. Wasserman 2012; *Fixed* 2013). In these ways, controversy surrounding the ethical ramifications of human enhancement implicates persons with disabilities practically as well as theoretically.

The philosophy of transhumanism and the goals and commitments of disability rights activism, at first, appear to coordinate. A key example is the fact that both points of view often reject the notion of species-typical functioning and accompanying normative judgments (Amundson 2000; Wasserman 2012, 5–6; Wolbring 2009; 192, cf. Daniels 1985). Wolbring asks how species-typical bodies are better when he claims that his mobility through crawling or using a chair is merely different—no better, no worse—than walking (*Fixed* 2013). Athlete and supermodel Aimee Mullins asks how species-typical bodies are better when she says: "People say I have no legs, but I say I have 10" (referring to her prosthetics, *Fixed* 2013). Bostrom asks how species-typical bodies are better when he notes that the human body up to now is mortal and open to injury and disease (e.g. 2007). Perhaps, then, the transhumanist's and the disability rights activist's interest in technological augmentation and innovation are much the same. Although transhumanists seek to improve the human body through augmentation, they do not immediately appear committed to judging persons with disabilities deficient in some special way. Rather, all human beings are treated as deficient for the transhumanist and can be improved (Wolbring 2008, 254; cf. Wasserman 2012). This may be appealing for members of the disability rights movement. Consider the aforementioned universalizing move some disability rights activists employ by using the term "Temporarily Able-Bodied" (TAB) to refer to those currently considered "abled," thereby dismissing the strong binary regularly constructed between ability and disability.

Further, contemporary experiences of disability are wedded to technology. Braille allows access for those with vision impairments. Prosthetics, hearing aids, communication assistants, speech-to-text and text-to-speech devices, converted vehicles, glucose meters, power chairs—all of these items and more are part of the landscape of disability. Access to evolving technologies is in many cases the bedrock for disability access and equality. But, the relationship between disability and technology runs deeper. The "things of disability" are so much a part of daily life that, for some, these technological objects become an extension of personal embodiment, the center of a "technological phenomenology" (Smit 2013). Tech-focused transhumanists are intrigued by these circumstances, which frame disabled persons as obvious allies in the move toward an increasingly technologized future. Transhumanist thinkers and those committed to enhancement projects thus invoke those in disability communities as representative of the forefront and potential of new technologies (Wasserman 2012).

But, a close investigation of the aims of disability rights and the suggested strategies of radical enhancement enthusiasts reveals that the two movements are significantly in tension with each other. Each imagines a different future for disability. Of course, communities of difference and disability are diverse, have a wide variety of needs and goals, and may often have discordant philosophies of political action. Yet, to borrow a formula from feminist philosophy, I claim that disability rights movements might at minimum agree that, first, ableism—widespread prejudicial treatment of persons with disabilities—exists; and, second, these circumstances must be changed. So, groups engaged in disability activism may disagree on why ableism exists, and what must be done to change it, but can be expected to aim toward the amelioration of ableism.

Therefore, the key question emerges: does transhumanism, as it is currently wielded by influential thinkers in bioethics, contribute to the goal of ameliorating ableism? And, would its preferred and recommended strategies of radical human enhancement contribute to this goal? In transhumanism's technological vision of the future, is there a place for disability? Transhumanist philosophers offer up specific programs and strategies of human enhancement, and their claims for a better world can only be evaluated by taking these specific strategies into view. In this book I considered a variety of transhumanist strategies, including the transcendence of embodiment and negative genetic selection. These strategies frame disability and embodied vulnerability more generally as risky while at the same time hypostasizing the notion of genetic deviance and the line between normality and abnormality. It is undeniable that technologies structure individual experiences of disability, and the proliferation and development of technology has played an integral role in the social movement toward disability equality. But, I have argued that transhumanist deployments of the importance and meaning of technology, especially reproductive technologies, positions disability as a risk to be managed, and, eventually, a thing to be eliminated.

Technology mediates experiences of disability in significant ways and marks off places and spaces of disability. Heightened access to social and political contexts for those with disabilities is tied to reliable and effective technologies of all kinds. Technology has set the stage for and advanced the disability rights movement in the United States and elsewhere. While technology plays an important role in disability rights activism, contra some enthusiasts, new technology alone will not radically reposition persons with disabilities in society. Emerging technologies must be paired with a revolution in values and concerted effort to dismantle the stigma surrounding disability.

If transhumanism encourages naturalization, materialization, and medicalization of disability, it is antithetical to disability rights movements as typically conceived. For instance, Harlan Lane sees the history of disability's construction and reception in social and political contexts running in parallel to that of marginalized sexual orientations; he notes that persons identified with both experienced three phases: "moral, medical and now social constructions" (2010, 78). As I outline in Chapter 3, disabilities were once considered moral issues and in connection with that were managed by the church and within the family; more commonly now disabilities are considered the domain of medical intervention and in connection that of interest for medicine. Meanwhile, disability rights movements treat disability as social and, at their best, do not use the word disability merely to refer to problems to be solved. With these things in mind, I challenge the potential of transhumanist visions for promoting projects of disability rights. In the remainder of this chapter, I consider issues connected to independence, vulnerability, and cognitive enhancement to support my challenge.

Independence and Vulnerability

Transhumanists believe new technologies should be welcomed as potentially improving human life, although they are risky (Bostrom 2005b, Garreau 2005, 115; Rubin 2008, 137). What individuals stand to gain, according to transhumanists, is the "use of technology to extend their mental and physical (including reproductive) capacities and to improve *their control over their own lives*" (Bostrom 2005b, Appendix, emphasis mine). In what feels like an echo, technology has provided greater possibilities for concerted political action and shaped rhetoric surrounding "independent living" for persons with disabilities. But, feminist disability scholars and philosophers of disability critique the rhetoric of independence in disability rights projects on the basis of its many exclusions.

Disability theorist Christine Kelly, for example, argues that disability activism has been unduly influenced by physically disabled white males, who focus on goals like independent living. According to Kelly, organizations like the U.S.-based ADAPT retain the echoes of this hidden identity of disability activism; she writes: "reinforcing independence as the ultimate social value is also a political act that maintains the status quo" (2010). ADAPT, she argues, assumes the superiority of the nuclear family and is heteronormative in the construction of the family. For an alternative idea of what disability activism aims for, consider disability theorist and activist Paul Longmore's words: "[activists] declare that they prize not self-sufficiency but self-determination, not independence but interdependence, not functional separateness but personal connection, not physical autonomy but human community" (quoted in Rohrer 2005, 36).

The transhumanist utopias I consider in this project are not only biologically but also politically outlined; for instance, Bostrom imagines a world of wide access to technologies and new political and moral possibilities which open up as a result of cognitive enhancement (Bostrom 2004, 2008). Traditional liberalism and transhumanism mimic each other by positing a fantasy subject that is *not* dependent and that can *choose* without limitation; this subject is rational and atomistic. This fantasy is detached from interpersonal realities and the contingencies of social and political life; the focus in both these discourses on atomism and individuality obscures fundamental human interdependence. In both locations—politics and bioethics—the disabled subject is constructed as uniquely dependent and limited, the correlative of the independent fantasy subject.

Autonomy in the liberal tradition is often reckoned in economic terms as the ability to earn wages. Nancy Fraser and Linda Gordon claim that dependency is connected to economic lives while at the same time having "pejorative" implications: "Informed by . . . general features of industrial-era semantics, a distinctive welfare-related use of *dependency* developed in the United States . . . this use of the term was fundamentally ambiguous, slipping easily, and repeatedly, from an economic meaning to a moral/psychological meaning" (2002, 22). Independence was and is ascribed to wage-earning members of the populace who are believed to have the ability to live autonomous lives and who thus escape the moral implications of dependence: "all dependency is suspect, and independence is enjoined upon everyone" (26). Martha Fineman also notes the economic tone in discourse about dependency. She argues that the "solutions" to problems of poverty and dependency often seem to include "paternity proceedings," along with child support that would partially reinstate the nuclear family. This, she argues, is meant to alleviate the difficulties presented by single motherhood to the economically sensitive relationship between the public and the private, normally obscured by carework inside the home (2002, 225). So, on her view, rhetorical touchstones of dependency, such as single mothers, showcase what is often at stake in these debates: gendered notions of the family and work.

Persons with disabilities are seen as "outliers" of the wage-earning community, in Anita Silvers' sense of "outlier."[5] They, unlike independent wage-earners, historically and presently require social support in order to continue to eat, live and work. Fineman helps challenge the "outlier" status of persons with disabilities and brings overblown praise of economic "autonomy" down to earth. Fineman elaborates the distinction between the public and the private (with the family as the locus) and its problematic relationship to vulnerability and dependency. She claims that notions of independence and autonomy are enabled by and supported through family work and care, which provides for its traditionally labeled "independent" and traditionally labeled "dependent" members in irreplaceable measure. In other words, the independent members of the household are freed from the household's day-to-day work and responsibilities in order to leave the home and become a wage-earner. The tasks of daily living (the maintenance of food, clothing, and shelter) are delegated to other members of the family, while at the same time benefiting the wage-earner (2002, 218).

Fineman is pointing toward the fundamental dependency at the root of independence; without the care work of the family, independence (as it is traditionally construed) would be impossible (2002, 215). Private labor is not aired in the social realm, however; instead, it is hidden behind political economy and official wages, receiving the attention of neither (216–8). This is how universal dependency is "masked." Usual definitions of autonomy and independence are based upon asymmetrical relationships represented by hidden private labor, and so reveal themselves as at least a partial myth. The ability to earn wages and be "fully cooperative" members of society can often "depend" upon the work of those construed as dependent (historically, the wife and children, who "belong" to the so-called family man).

So, the independence of the wage-earning class is illusory and fundamentally dependent upon unpaid carework accomplished in the private sphere. This insight calls into question the value of "autonomy" itself, as it is typically construed—especially in opposition to dependence. As Fineman argues, the fundamental dependency of all members of liberal, democratic society is *masked* through the bright line drawn between dependency and independence and the relegation in the public imagination of all neediness to the oppressed and vulnerable. In a complex analysis of political economy and social alienation, disability theorist James Charlton theorizes that "backward attitudes about disability are not the basis for disability oppression, disability oppression is the basis for backward attitudes" (2010, 151). In other words, the disability oppression that cuts persons with disabilities from economic and social life gives rise to stigmatizing attitudes. In turn, these stigmatizing attitudes stifle efforts to rise up against disability oppression. Charlton writes: "Instead of curing the social conditions that cause disease and desperation . . . the dominant culture explains the pitiful conditions people are forced to live in by creating a stratum or group of 'naturally' pitiful individuals to conceal its pitiful status quo. The dominant culture turns reality on its head" (2010, 156). Ultimately, neither dependence nor independence is natural, but both are treated as such and the social conditions which construct these subject positions are hidden away. As a result, persons with disabilities internalize stigmatizing attitudes and see themselves as separate from, and more dependent than, others. They are psychically alienated:

> Most people with disabilities actually come to believe they are less normal, less capable than others. Self-pity, self-hate, shame, and other manifestations of this process are devastating for they prevent people with disabilities from knowing their real selves, their real needs, and their real capabilities and from recognizing the options they in fact have. (Charlton 2010, 151)

All of this, according to Charlton, stands in the way of disability rights movements and maintains disability oppression.

Disability rights projects should, then, call for radical economic reconstruction and involve conceptual work revising notions of autonomy and dependency in a way that attends carefully to the nuances of interdependent living and the reality of universal dependency and neediness. While no one should be denied housing, calls for independent living are not enough for disability rights projects. That means transhumanist fantasies of control through technology are linked to an exclusionary form of disability politics that fails to question the deep social and economic circumstances that create oppression. Calls for the recognition of complex networks of interdependence (networks in which all persons are engaged) should replace calls for independence and control.

Along these lines, I call for a radical rethinking of what counts as "enhancement." We must "enhance" our acceptance of our own dependency and vulnerability and refuse the rhetorical system by which persons with disabilities are alone considered dependent. Feminist ethics of care is controversial in feminist circles and in disability studies, but work in this area can help us begin rethinking autonomy, dependence, and disability.

Key to the discourse of the "ethics of care" is the contention that autonomy, rendered in traditional liberal theory as accomplishing key acts without significant assistance, must be replaced or transformed as the central characteristic of personhood (Kittay 2001, 570). This theory is geared toward recognizing the flaws in common notions of both autonomy and dependency. Theorists like Eva Kittay wish to recast the role of the "dependent"—including individuals with disabilities—and open up space for a responsive ethic (570). Tied to this aim is that of recasting the role of the care-giver and providing social support to them in an attempt to mitigate the impact of biased views of the meaning of that support (573). "Justice as caring" is the expression of the responsive ethic that Kittay outlines.

Kittay and her partner were already committed academics at the time she gave birth to her daughter, Sesha. Upon discovering that Sesha would not share in what Kittay and her partner most valued, Kittay began to undergo a reorientation in her thinking which allowed the recognition of Sesha's life as valuable and connected to her own unique conception of the good. Kittay criticizes liberal notions of personhood for being unable to treat her daughter as a citizen of any country (2001, 567) or as a subject of justice (574) or as a person (568). In other words, traditional liberalism excludes Sesha, as does traditional bioethics. Kittay finds this unbearable and counter-intuitive (558).

Kittay writes: "constructed only as a problem, Sesha and other developmentally disabled persons appear to have no claim to the aids and supports that they need to live and live well" (2001, 567). For Kittay, "being a person has little to do with rationality and everything to do with relationships to our world and to those in it" (568). Kittay argues that liberal notions of personhood must be overhauled in light of this recognition. On her view of justice as caring, "being a person means having the capacity to be in certain relationships with other persons, to sustain contact with other persons, to shape one's own world and the world of others, and to have a life that another person can conceive of as an imaginative possibility for him or herself" (568). For Kittay, it is clear that Sesha fulfills these criteria of personhood. She enjoys music and laughter and the people she knows and loves. On Kittay's view, focusing on her deficiency is unjust, and "only by considering her in the fullness of her joys and capacities can we view her impairments in light of her life, her interests, her happiness—and not as projections of her 'able' parents or of an able-biased society." But, it is only through the appropriate social support for care and care workers, along with social support for Sesha herself, will help expose the fullness of her personhood and allow focus to be reoriented away from Sesha's differences (Kittay 2001, 567). As Charlton would remind us, disability oppression as lack of social support feeds stigmatizing attitudes.

For Kittay, "justice as caring" can open up the opportunity for society to support diverse ways of living. She writes: "those who have developmental disabilities require more supports than those without these impairments. However, they also provide different and rich opportunities for relationships and experiencing new ways of seeing the world" (2001, 567). This outcome, however, is threatened by society's bias against dependence. On Kittay's view, independence is a "fiction," which

> turns those whose dependence cannot be masked into pariahs, or makes them objects of disdain or pity. It causes us to refuse assistance when it is needed. It encourages us either to deny that assistance to others when they require it or to be givers of care because we fear having to receive care ourselves. In acknowledging dependency, we respect the fact that as individuals our dependency relations are constitutive of who we are and that, as a society, we are inextricably dependent on one another. (2001, 570)

For Kittay, then, an overhaul of the liberal conception of personhood is required. The over-emphasis on rationality in that context, she argues, is problematic because it leaves out significantly vulnerable populations and denies them justice rightly deserved (2001, 562–5). For Kittay, social interdependence renders us all vulnerable, and it would be a mistake of hubris to forget or deny "the dependent animals we are" (2001, 576).

But dependence is precisely what transhumanists want to forget and repeatedly bemoan; more specifically, transhumanists seek to transcend the vulnerability of embodiment, and the rhetoric used to promote this transcendence links disability in a special way with vulnerability. Bostrom believes most people are culpably complacent with regard to humanity's worst problems—especially the problem of human mortality, which he claims costs us access to invaluable knowledge (2007). For him, the body is fragile, and parents have a responsibility to leave their children with better "homes" (2010). This focus on knowledge and denigration of the vulnerability of the human body exposes the dualism between mind and body at the heart of transhumanism, and the accompanying desire to protect the mind from the body. The transhumanist envisions a mind released from the body, and therefore seeks the transcendence of embodiment—mind without body is transhumanism's posthuman. Many with disabilities seek wider acceptance of the melding of body and machine in novel and surprising ways—the better to release lived experiences of disability from the stranglehold of stigma and achieve the aims of everyday living—but these goals are not the same as the goal of transcendence.

Mitigating the stigma of disability requires rejecting the problematic social and cultural reception of dependence and embracing embodiment in its vulnerability. Disability theorist Ruth Hubbard writes: "People shun persons who have disabilities and isolate them so they will not have to see them. They fear them as though the disability were contagious. And it is, in the sense that it forces us to face our own vulnerability" (2010, 107).

Cognitive Enhancement

While the alliance between transhumanists and persons with physical disabilities who use assistive technologies regularly seems at least plausible, any possible alliance between transhumanists and persons with cognitive differences is difficult to imagine. Throughout this book, issues connected with cognitive ability have continually arisen. As previously discussed, Bostrom seeks to protect the mind from the body, and enshrines cognitive capacity as key to the good life. Indeed, when he decries the fact of mortality, he frames the death of others as a loss quantifiable in terms of the number of books the person who died might have written—that is, in terms of lost knowledge (2007). In a paper co-authored with Anders Sandberg on cognitive enhancement, Bostrom and Sandberg begin with the following assumption:

> There are few resources more useful than cognitive ability. While other resources are necessary or desirable, cognition enables them to be used for achieving personal goals. While there is little evidence that high intelligence causes happiness there appears to be ample evidence that low intelligence increases the risk for accidents, negative life events, and low income (Gottfredson 1997, 2004) while higher intelligence promotes health (Whalley and Deary 201) and wealth. (2006, 201)

Notice again the linkage of disability, this time cognitive difference, with risk, along with the lack of attention to social, cultural, and political factors that might explain the correlations described.

Existing transhumanist projects maintain existing hierarchies among capabilities by linking capability with well-being. For transhumanists, the greater the number of capabilities, the larger the opportunity range, the better the life.

Philosophers of disability, contra transhumanists, have worked to disentangle well-being from capability and argue that the lack of a capability should not be assumed to diminish well-being (e.g. Asch 2003, 318). One way to fight ableism is to deny that difference must signal deficiency, and that the lack of a particular capability reliably lessens quality of life. Transhumanists cling to the intellect as the most fundamental of capabilities, but fighting ableism and promoting an inclusive disability rights program absolutely requires a radical reexamination of the privileged position of the intellect.

Transhumanists and enhancement enthusiasts alike assume that a better future—that is, a more just, more moral future—turns on the possibility of improved intellects (Bostrom 2008). They assume increased cognitive capacity for individuals would bring about better social conditions for all persons (as described in Koch 2010). Savulescu, who promotes genetic selection as the most efficient mode of enhancement, emphasizes the importance of selecting for any gene which may impact intellectual capacity (even if the connection between gene and outcome is only suspected or is unclear) (e.g. 2001b). James Hughes frames transhumanism in terms of a "struggle for a smarter world" (2008). It is abundantly clear, then, that transhumanists intend to ally themselves only with *some* disabled persons; their recommendations regarding cognitive capacity trade on widespread rejection of those with cognitive difference and reveal their investment in eliminating disability.

Rethinking notions of autonomy and independence involves rethinking the special stigma against and lack of concern for persons with cognitive differences. Leslie Francis aids the project of reworking autonomy by pointing to its collaborative nature. In her own words, she wants to "destabilize some aspects" of the idea that "people with intellectual disabilities . . . lack autonomy, at least if their disabilities are significantly severe" (2009, 200). She notes some reasons why this idea is common: "Some people with intellectual disabilities have difficulty with abstract reasoning. Others have difficulty with impulse control. Still others may have difficulty in planning ahead and in pursuing developed plans" (204). Limitations in "social adaptation" also present some issues, like "gullibility, naïveté, and the risk of victimization" (204). Generally, a variety of models for the mind can "agree on the presence of some kind of executing processing system" that is often lacking among those with cognitive disabilities (204–5). Yet, Francis points out that tools necessary for enhancing physical functioning (i.e. her examples of eyeglasses and cars) are not considered illustrative of the lack of physical autonomy on the part of users; perhaps, then, tools necessary for enhancing intellectual functioning need not be so, either. On her view: "The point is that what it is for 'me' to do something—whether it requires certain skills that I exercise independently, for example—is at least partially a matter of the context and goals of the activity" (205). Dependence and collaboration, even among those with cognitive differences, does not preclude substantial quality of life.

Francis argues that "conceptions of the good can be individually tailored and rooted in individual psychological states without being arrived at independently" (2009, 206). She notes that persons considered autonomous—and therefore happy—are fundamentally dependent in a variety of ways, including on friends and family; we rely on others like Ulysses, who used "ropes and masts [as] prosthetic devices . . . in his effort to resist the sirens" who tempted him to fling himself to his death (207). Francis further argues that there are substantial non-cognitive elements in relationships and collaboration and that "ordinary individuals have interests in what happens to them, and they have interests in the interests of others; persons with intellectual disabilities have these interests as well" (211). For Francis, "people come to understand their interests in interconnection with others" (*ibid.*, cf. Meyer 2005)

Transhumanism's pernicious attitude with regard to the absolute value of cognition upholds ableism and dualism between the body and the mind. Members of the disability community demand respect that can only be expressed through a strategy of acceptance: embracing or celebrating disability as only one part of persons whose "lives—impairments and all—are respectable, acceptable ways to live" (Asch 2000b, 243; cf. Silvers 2009).

CONCLUSION

A sustained critique of the promotion of genetic selection as a strategy of enhancement is of vital importance. It can expand issues of reproductive choice to those of reproductive justice and attend to the normalization attendant upon prenatal testing practices. In the preceding pages, I continued my consideration of the role of genetic determinism in discourse regarding medical interventions. I used the notion of genetic determinism in a restatement of the Adrienne Asch's disability critique and I strengthened the critique through a renewed focus on institutions and social conditions. In the course of my discussion, I defended the original disability critique against the objection that it aims to curtail reproductive liberty. Further, I made a case against the possibility of transhumanist allies in disability rights projects.

To complete my critique of enhancement thinking, in the next chapter I discuss fields of risk posed by genetic selection practices and the participation of genetic counseling discourse in a system of actuarial thinking (a term I borrow from Dorothy Nelkin and Susan Lindee, 1995) and biopolitical decision-making that calls upon potential parents to perform autonomy as defined by risk-aversion. The potentially impaired fetus becomes a site of risk in this system. Ultimately, I describe transhumanism's desired subject as the disabled or deviant body's opposite. If biology is figured as destiny, it is easy to maintain a false binary between abled and disabled, or between a realm of pure choice and a dangerous realm of pure chance and risk (here, genetic chance and fetal risk). As we have seen, transhumanist logic rejects the disabled body as limiting choice and describes a selected or enhanced body as enjoying access to a realm of pure choice. On this view, choosing to utilize evolving technology in the arena of genetic selection can multiply freedom and choice and therefore unlock better futures. On my view, genetic selection, as an enhancement technique, merely serves to enhance stigma and fear connected to risk and disability—it does not enhance human life.

NOTES

1. Interestingly, Savulescu mentions that the pursuit of equality among minorities is one good reason to support procreative autonomy against procreative beneficence. But, he argues that equality should be dealt with politically and socially rather than through reproductive means (2001b, 425). I argue that the same should be said of enhancement.

2. As noted in the introduction and Chapter 2, I do not mean this phrase to refer to embryos or fetuses.

3. For an excellent sustained critique of the idea that the good life involves a multiplicity of choices, see Claudia Mills, "The Child's Right to an Open Future?" (2003). Significant choice is an important part of life; but the mere proliferation of choice is not necessary for a good life and at times the pursuit of options can impede a good life.

4. Parents whose newborn or infant children have a fatal condition request strongly that on-site medical professionals call their children by their given names (personal correspondence in April 2012 with Donna Patno, a nurse at the Cleveland Clinic Fetal Care Center in Ohio). We can understand this as a reaction to naming via diagnosis.

5. "Theories of justice often fasten on specific differences in people's attainment of whatever intrinsic or instrumental value(s) the particular theory embraces. Individuals who are value-deficient because they cannot rise to or instantiate the property(ies) the theory picks out as valuable, or who are reservoirs of properties the theory picks out as disvalues, are likely to be portrayed as outliers" (Silvers 2009, 174).

Chapter 5

Disability as/at Risk

The Biopolitics of Disability

The linkage of disability and risk in transhumanist literature, in discourses surrounding reproductive technology, and in popular media puts those with disabilities at mortal risk. In other words, the very desire transhumanists, bioethics literature, and biomedical contexts express to eliminate risk paradoxically produces and assigns risk to particular persons. Meanwhile, claims regarding the special relationship between risk and disability are spurious. The practice of risk management, whether theoretical or actual, redoubles risk; envisioning a utopia without risk creates risky techniques that literally kill and victimize particular persons.

Part of what is at stake in this chapter is the exploration of the biopolitical discourse of responsible subjectivity as a choice-maker against risk. Foucault's discussion of biopower engages power not just as a negative, but also as a positive, phenomenon—so too can we trace the differential impact of practices like genetic counseling and the ways in which it serves as an organ of biopower. In the milieu of genetic counseling, parents are asked to express their subjectivity as risk managers and particular populations become managed populations, marked in the womb as the bearers of contagious risk.

Bioethics literature more largely is riddled with suggestions regarding the characteristics of the responsible medical subject. This responsible subject is a choice-maker, risk-averse and thoughtful, who plans for contingencies and successfully wields the power of attorney and pen. We are urged to set up bulwarks against personal risks by creating Ulysses contracts (contracts that hold even if we change our minds) and Advanced Directives (contracts that hold if we can no longer express our wishes) so that we can "die with dignity" and control the treatments we undergo even when we are unconscious or confused. In response, we seek to stretch our agency into time and space and crave control, especially control over a future self who may be in a different mindset. Meanwhile, when we decide to reproduce, we are urged to meet with genetic counselors and discuss the likely attributes and quality of life of our progeny so that we can make "informed decisions" regarding how, when, and who to reproduce. Again, these processes are posed as risk assessment and parents are urged to be choice-makers even prior to the initiation of pregnancy. Parents are urged to create the best child possible, which most often means choosing not to produce other children whose embodiment is conceptually connected with risk and vulnerability.

In his work, Foucault pinpoints the development of normalizing practices (discursive, institutional, and otherwise)—which distinguish between normal and abnormal subjects. In bioethics discourse, the responsible medical subject is the normal subject who chooses against risk. This normal subject is set up against the risky embodiment of others; these others are viewed as "abnormal" insofar as they are subject to chance and are seen as threats to the entire community. The responsible medical subject is also the responsible citizen. In this context, bodies, populations, and countries are spaces or canvases of exclusion, regulation and risk. Again, the eye of biopolitics rests here upon the "species body" and the enhancement of that body, in a deeply dynamic and fully participatory framework of contamination and exclusion.

GENETIC COUNSELING AND DISABILITY AS RISK

I turn now to directly analyze genetic counseling and how it presents genetic information and makes this information operational in decision-making—that is, a part of responsible parenting. Genetic counseling is a key part of the medical and cultural context of genetic selection. In the United States, genetic counselors can be genetic experts, physicians or other medical professionals (Davis 2010, 5). Or, they can be specifically trained through graduate study in accessing, presenting and interpreting genetic testing, earning a Master's degree and certification by the American Board of Genetic Counseling ("KidsHealth" 2012). Genetic counselors assist individuals curious about their own genotype and family history or who seek information during the reproductive decision-making process.

Genetic counseling may also occur much less formally, as through the data provided by private companies like 23andMe, which offer at-home testing kits. 23andMe has been touted as a way to "help you manage risk and make informed decisions" (23andMe 2013). This service, in addition to its $199 at-home testing kit, offers interactive tools to share one's information and collects survey data to link to the genetic data it collects.[1] Sonia Gawel, a satisfied customer whose endorsement appeared on 23andMe's homepage early in its development, wrote that the company is "seriously amazing! Learning so much about my genetics/disease risk/traits, etc. Now I can design my lifestyle for prevention!" (review posted to website June 26, 2012). In other words, the genetic data Gawel received from the company may allow her to interpret the risk posed by certain activities on an individual level (a healthy diet and exercise may help alleviate the genetic predisposition to cardiovascular disease) and bring information about her traits to the table when the time comes to reproduce.

Genetic counseling in formal settings is ruled by multiple strong norms of professional conduct. I discuss two of the most important norms here. First, genetic counselors reportedly value and seek to maintain the autonomy of their clients above all else, a fact which Dena Davis claims is easily explained by a handful of factors, including awareness of the threat of coercion (informed by cultural knowledge of eugenic history) and the fact that many consider reproductive decision-making to be an extremely private affair (1997, 7 and 2010, 13–17). Second, genetic counselors are committed to nondirective counseling, as stated in the Code of Ethics of the National Society of Genetic Counselors (quoted in Davis 1997, 8). Nondirective counseling is articulated by the profession as the presentation of facts and the exploration and realization of parental values without interference or input stemming from counselor values or outside influence (quoted Davis 1997, 8).

I claim that there are two helpful ways to read the concept of choice (and, therefore, autonomy) in the arena of genetic counseling. First, using the work of Anne Waldschmidt, which in turn engages a Foucauldian frame, I consider the production of an autonomous subject who can choose to avoid risk ("Now I can design my lifestyle for prevention!"). Second, I consider Dena Davis' argument that the choice parents enjoy with regard to reproduction is at times trumped by children's rights to a future autonomy, an *open future*. Exploring the play of choice in these two ways will allow us to uncover the mythos of the disabled body as a site of risk, and the unmarked or abled body as a site of choice. This leads me to the conclusion that in the biopolitical logic, the disabled and abled bodies are figured as opposites. I also describe the way in which the fetus is presented as a site of risk—an *impaired fetus* to women or partner reproducers. I conclude that the milieu of prenatal testing and genetic counseling is a realm that *enhances* the concepts of risk and disability, but fails to enhance quality of life.

Anne Waldschmidt's essay "Who is Normal? Who is Deviant?" brings the practice and influence of genetic counseling into view through a Foucauldian framework of governmentality (Waldschmidt 2005). Foucault's work, again, is meant to capture the operation of normalizing influences in the creation of the subject and the boundaries and character of subjectivity. In the case of genetic counseling, "risk management" becomes the management of the subject and the development of the roles of parent, impaired fetus, and "value-free" counseling in a network of actuarial thinking.

Waldschmidt insists on a distinction between "normativity" and "normality," arguing that normativity "refers to the power of social and legal norms that are imposed upon people" while normality "involves comparing people with each other in light of a standard" (2005, 193). While the former no longer has great purchase in neoliberal societies which focus upon autonomy, the latter appears and operates in "data-oriented societies" (194). Statistical data comparing subjects has a tight relationship with norms; "evaluations and expectations" (notice: not "value judgments") tag along after statistics themselves are crunched and publicized (194). Foucault frames statistics as a field generated by the interests of biopower (Foucault 2003b, 250; Lemke 2011, 5).

Again, the contemporary field of genetic counseling relies fundamentally upon the principle of client (parent) autonomy, which is upheld through non-directive counseling (Davis 1997, 8). According to Waldschmidt, the practice maintains governing force over clients through normality. Genetic counseling presents medical, hereditary, and age-related statistics along with risk of deviation and associated costs to the potential parents and requires decisive action in response to those statistics. "Evaluations and expectations" are communicated and comparisons within the population are produced, but no value judgments are expressed by the counselor. The counselor expects the potential or actual reproducer to express their autonomy by taking action, and the expected action which best expresses autonomy in this context necessarily involves removing oneself from a field of perceived risk or protecting oneself against risk in some way (Waldschmidt 2005, 205). Not acting upon received genetic information can be seen as an immoral refusal to exercise autonomy. Risk transforms the counseled individuals into specific subjects: autonomous subjects who can choose against "misfortune" by utilizing the platform of "statistical calculation" (204–205; cf. Morrison 2008).

In a hypothetical situation built from counseling experience, genetic counselor Dena Davis presents a case of risk communication and decision-making carried out between counselors and an older, relatively uninformed couple, Missie and Hank. Medical experts had determined from ultrasounds that the fetus Missie was carrying likely had spina bifida, a condition encompassing a range of impacts (2010, 9). While the experts were unsure whether the fetus would have spina bifida and were also unsure about how severe such the impact of this condition would be, Missie sought certainty. Remember, here, Carlson's prenatal prototypes, which are taken as guiding even when fundamentally indeterminate.

Davis reports that "the counselors, among themselves, had agreed that it was probably in Missie's best interest to abort. They had a 'gut sense' that the fetus was damaged, despite the slight chance that it was healthy" (2010, 10). After asking without success for more information, Missie told them: "Okay, I'll do whatever you tell me. Tell me what to do" (10). In response, "the counselors gently but firmly declined" to give Missie direction, and so eventually she made an appointment for an abortion, which the counselors considered provisional until Missie confirmed it from home (10). Despite Missie's repeatedly expressed desperation for advice, the counselors refused to provide it, instead communicating only statistics and the prenatal prototype. Missie used this information to make her decision, which the counselors believed they had safeguarded as autonomous by way of the communication of only statistics in compliance with their norm of non-directive counseling.

To analyze the context of Missie's decision, note that Missie was to absorb the possibility of risk and respond to it in an expression of (highly individualized) autonomy. She sought to connect personally with others in the context of her decision-making but was refused for fear of interrupting her autonomy. Waldschmidt evaluates the role of risk in communication between genetic counselors and potential mothers. She argues that the concept and deployment of risk establishes a gloss of neutrality and objectivity in genetic counseling, thus obviating the need for counselors to give "explicit advice" to mothers but still communicating a specific message about appropriate action (2005, 204). She argues that contrary to common perceptions of objectivity, statistical data developed regarding risks are constructed in highly contingent ways and can be expressed in a variety of forms which have predictable affective impacts on the individual to whom they are communicated (199–203). Her argument is supported by the narratives of women who are given or who have sought genetic counseling (Parens and Asch, 2000, 7; see also Saxton 2000).

Further, according to Waldschmidt, "risk" attaches itself to bodies (fetuses and mothers) through the practice of prenatal diagnostics (2005, 197). She calls this the "individualization of risk" and argues that it operates as a "normalizing technique" in the case of decision-making (198). Autonomous and individualized decision-making, the goal of genetic counseling, is a complex process of situating oneself alongside or within a range of statistical normality and participating in the avoidance or management of risk. She writes: "In the past, experts could give direct advice; in the days of neoliberal government, however, they may only help clients to identify their own positions in the broad terrain of normality and deviation" (198). Sonia Gawel's endorsement of 23andMe testifies to this focus on risk when Gawel equates risk with genetic data itself, enthusing that she is: "Learning so much about my genetics/disease risk/traits, etc." Gawel takes up the role of risk management when she writes: "Now I can design my lifestyle for prevention!"

So, the body is a site of risk, and risk is most often interpreted as dangerous threat by those who encounter it or are told they may be susceptible to it.

Any predisposition or tested trait deviating from a norm within a population becomes a risk and marks the body through prenatal diagnostics. Disabled embodiment—and even the bodies of mothers themselves, who should undergo genetic counseling even without any prior indications—becomes inherently risky, a dangerous threat. Recall that the newest diagnostic testing procedures merely compare fetal DNA to DNA from a presumptively normal person who stands in for a canonical genotype. Any deviance is risk—tracking individual linkages between genotype and trait becomes unnecessary.

Increasingly, at-home genetic testing kits (direct-to-consumer, or DTC kits) are being made available. The availability and marketing of these kits highlights the focus on autonomy and privacy that is made so paramount within the field of genetic counseling. It also represents an effort to provide individuals with as much data as possible so they can participate in autonomous decision-making, especially with regard to reproduction. But, to the contrary, Waldschmidt shows that the communication of statistical risk governs and normalizes the subject, which means that this increasing individualization and privacy promotes autonomy only on the surface. Continuing emphasis on individual choice and the proliferation of individualized data regarding genetics obscures the pointed goals of testing and screening. Genetic data is meant to provide individuals with tools toward ends already specified in medical and popular culture. These ends are the avoidance or elimination of certain conditions, seen through the imperfect (partial) lens of genotype.

Prenatal prototypes are here made operational. According to Waldschmidt:

> statistics and prognoses are presented to real people, people who face real decisions and constraints—women who must quickly decide whether they wish to carry an unborn child to term, or abort it. And, of course, the normality-risk concept and the entire (insurance) setting within which the risk is presented do not allow any doubt about what kind of decision is expected from the individual woman: the decision not to have a child with a congenital impairment. (2005, 205)

Waldschmidt exposes the value system at the root of the "facts" of heredity and genetic statistical risk. Employing the norms of genetic counseling requires a strong distinction between facts and values, but this distinction is unfounded. Remember the gut instincts held by the genetic counselors in Missie's case. Genetic data as presented in counseling sessions is anything but value-free and nondirective. Risk, used to communicate complex statistics, is a concept with affective resonance. It presents the probable or potential end state as a dangerous threat to be avoided, even when this characterization is unjustified.

Beyond acceptance that deviance is to be avoided, there is little significant reflection about what conditions should be targeted and what tests are important to develop and invest in.[2] The most frequently screened condition, Down syndrome, is targeted again and again as an undesirable condition, and yet is not fatal or necessarily painful. Nemours, a pediatric medical system with hospitals in several states, maintains a website focused on children's health which provides information regarding genetic counseling for curious parents. This resource has the following advice to offer potential parents: "Experts recommend that all pregnant women, regardless of age or circumstance, be offered genetic counseling and testing to screen for Down syndrome" ("KidsHealth" 2012). Justification for this recommendation is not provided. And misleading statistics and outdated information regarding the cost of raising a child with Down syndrome have been used in recent years. For example, potential parents have been advised that their child may be either relatively typical cognitively or severely cognitively limited. This poses the chances of severe cognitive limitation as if it were fifty-percent. But, in reality, the chances of severe cognitive limitation for a person with genetic indication for Down syndrome are below 5 percent (Elkins and Brown 1995, 18 cited in Carlson 2002, 209). In fact, according to Carlson, "seventy-five to ninety percent of persons with Down syndrome are capable of living independently of their families and are employable as adults" (2002, 209).

Procreative beneficence à la Julian Savulescu could be brought forward as one strategy useful for reflection about what conditions to target and the avoidance of repeated prejudices. But, as I have already argued, this principle is laced with genetic bias and also fails to remedy the issue of repeated and reinforced existing prejudice. Procreative beneficence will consistently recommend to a potential reproducer that the best choice is to have a child who will be favored in existing society. Savulescu acknowledges this result, but as aforementioned denies that such choices would likely produce significant inequality (defined, it seems, by population count) and if the choices did do so, procreative beneficence would suggest that new choices be made (2001b, 423).

Savulescu does argue (as noted in Chapter 4) that improving social life through tackling social inequalities and prejudices should not be attempted by way of reproductive decision-making, but this statement seems to contradict his overall perspective given that he attempts to improve individual lives through reproductive decision-making (2001b, 423). Surely it begs credulity for Savulescu to argue that he means this "improvement" to have no effect beyond the individual level. And, if his interest in individual improvement is not informed by social conditions, then it is cause for even greater concern—he fails to recognize the importance of social conditions for happiness.

Another conceptual option that might assist in the determination of what tests and screening procedures should be developed is the aforementioned "right to an open future" first promulgated by Joel Feinberg in 1980.

The "right to an open future" is a bundle of rights that includes rights held "in trust"—those that a child cannot yet exercise, but which should be protected for future use (1980, 125). Examples include the exercise of religion, thought to be the arena of adults, or reproductive rights. This bundle of rights is meant to ensure future autonomy and, therefore, an adult life with the most options or opportunities to articulate and pursue various versions of the good life. Translated into a genetic sense, violations of the right to an open future could include refusing to test for certain disease or non-disease traits, or choosing to create a child with what might be considered a limitation or risk. While Savulescu, as a utilitarian, does not endorse rights frameworks, Savulescu's procreative beneficence is meant to preclude precisely these sorts of problems.

Dena Davis picks up on this concept; she believes that genetic counselors and doctors should continue to respect parental autonomy in counseling settings, but also asserts that respect and protection of autonomy must not stop there (1997 e.g. 7–8, and 2010). Davis argues that a child's future autonomy must also be respected and protected, and that sometimes concerns for the child must trump the strong norms of value-free information and nondirective counseling. Davis asserts that genetic counselors are rightly troubled when potential parents may deliberately seek what most consider the risks of reproduction: deafness, for example, or hereditary Achondroplasia (1997, 8). Specifically, she considers the dilemma posed to genetic counselors in the case of Deaf parents who wish to select for a deaf child and would potentially reject a "healthy" child.

Davis worries that "elevating respect for patient autonomy above all other values" may make it "difficult to give proper weight to other factors, such as human suffering" and would perhaps be misleading in this case (1997, 7). She wants to reintroduce "space in which to give proper attention to the moral claims of the future child" (7). Davis reframes the issue at hand, whether or not it is wrong to deliberately create a deaf child, as pitting "parental autonomy" against the "child's future autonomy" (8). In this case, she believes that the child's future autonomy is the most important factor and the value-free counseling that genetic counselors usually employ should be abandoned. The genetic counselor should refuse to help the Deaf parents.

Yet, in line with what I have argued so far, this assumes that "the right to an open future" is the purview of the abled body, a body which becomes the imagined site of undetermined choice. It is as if the open future is chosen and the closed future is discarded when one chooses negative genetic selection. This logic works only if one indulges in genetic determinism and believes that prenatal prototypes, or single traits, give fully flowered information regarding a future child. This logic of the "spreading effect" also operates on the basis of a hierarchy between abled and disabled bodies—the marked body will always have a "more closed" future on this view, a presumption that is untenable. Some may venture that a child with Down syndrome will have fewer opportunities than a "neurotypical" child; but, even this assertion meets with difficulty. Any particular child with Down syndrome could have more opportunities and pleasures than any particular neurotypical child, because opportunities and pleasures are structured by social reception, which can be hostile or welcoming. The "right to an open future," translated in the genetic sense while disregarding social factors, leads one to behave as though disability is equal to limitation and unmarked or abled bodies are the privileged site of choice.

The woman or potential parent is constructed by the field of genetic counseling and the availability of prenatal diagnostics as a "risk manager"—an autonomous agent who responds to and manages risk. But, following Waldschmidt, these processes and practices risk attaches to bodies themselves. For instance, the woman's body becomes risky when she undergoes testing for genetic traits she may pass on to offspring. Furthermore, the fetus is the primary site of risk in these schemes. A new discursive category—the "impaired fetus" (the defective fetus) is brought into focus and augmented by these practices and innovations in these practices. While strong social models of disability tend to separate impairment and disability (in an echo of the construction of sex and gender) in order to argue that disability is socially constructed while impairment is not, it is important to notice that here impairment is socially constructed via the establishment of the fetus as a site of risk and deviance (Tremain 2006).[3]

Prenatal testing and selection strategies are not an enhancement strategy for individuals, as transhumanists imagine. Instead, they focus on statistical improvement across a population, and related discourse and practices merely "enhance" notions of risk and notions of disability—that is, they amp them up, attach them with increased meaning, and link their management to the expression of reproductive autonomy in medical contexts. Extensive modes of normalization attend these practices. Autonomy is expressed by asking the question: what makes a livable life? And answering: a life without risk.

I can now name a central feature of utopian, enhanced futures: a chosen subject, selected because it is not marked by disability and so is thought to be impervious to chance. In the general case, utopian thinking obscures the present state of affairs by wishing fervently for a non-existing state of affairs, a non-place. Transhumanist utopian thinking focuses on a subject that is not real, a fantastic subject; that is, a techno-liberal subject that experiences proliferating choice. The most pernicious feature of transhumanist utopian thinking is that the non-existent subject obscures and devalues the lives of already-existing persons. It wishes fervently for a subject whose absolute autonomy is ensured via choice-making mediated through technology. To the transhumanist, embodiment appears as inherently risky and undesirable.

The limitations of embodiment are made objects of fear in transhumanist thinking, and we frantically self-regulate in response to disciplinary and regulatory practices under a regime of biopower.

Davis justifies choosing children in prenatal diagnostic and negative selection contexts through "the right to an open future." But, no person can have an unencumbered and *individual* right to an open future, because such a thing would imply that chance plays no role and an absolute proliferation of choice is available to that individual. Inhabiting an open future is the underlying goal of enhancement, and the vision is created without reference to holding a future *in common*, open because we can be in control of it together. The transhumanist version of utopia is peopled by subjects autonomous in that they are *undetermined by others*—but mediated by technology, that is, techno-liberal subjects. Transhumanists seek this kind of absolute freedom, chosen and controlled individually.

In this vein, parents are urged to make choices in order to ensure the choice-making capability of their future children—that is, unencumbered space for individual autonomy. In other words, they are asked to determine what child they will have so that the child will be undetermined. Popular focus in bioethics on "designer children" obfuscates the point, since focusing on the "designed" character of progeny cannot capture the overarching quest for non-determination. There is a move here from urging reproducers to seek comparatively enhanced choice-making capabilities in future children (better, more, greater, most opportunity) to urging reproducers to seek an absolute choice-making character for their future child ensuring that child will experience no interference from chance. For the transhumanist, in order to achieve this end, the risks of embodiment must be subverted through reproductive choice-making. Choice-making is both the goal and the means of enhancement. To control the future and force it "open," the transhumanist must absolutely determine it and attempt to preclude determination from any other source (anything or anyone else). The future is open to me when it is chosen by me.

Disability traits are read by both Bostrom and Savulescu as risks—possible limitations on future freedoms. The transhumanist subject, by contrast, must be one that engenders no risks. A body carrying a disability trait, then, is this subject's opposite; it is viewed purely as risk through genetic counseling and figured as avoidable determination. Traits that can be screened in utero are seen as limiting; the future for the "impaired" fetus is imagined as a history already written—the transhumanists close this future. Un-enhanced bodies, then, seem to be locked in a field of risk. In sum, transhumanists seek to improve life through biotechnology. But, the notion transhumanists have of improvement is rooted in utopia, specifically a utopian subject: the techno-liberal individual. This is, of course, an overly narrow and exacting version of what a good and fulfilling life looks like. The choice for the techno-liberal subject is a biopolitical choice against certain kinds of bodies in the hope of improving life—under biopower, and in transhumanist literature, positive and negative eugenics are paired together. The transhumanists make a biological reduction while at the same time attempting to transcend the physical.

DISABILITY AT RISK

Foucault notes that under biopower, death takes multiple forms: "When I say 'killing,' I obviously do not mean simply murder as such, but also every form of indirect murder: the fact of exposing someone to death, increasing the risk of death for some people, or, quite simply, political death, expulsion, rejection, and so on" (2000b, 256). My primary motivation for writing this book is the insidious ways in which persons with disabilities are placed at risk by dominant discourses, unfortunately supported in bioethics, which devalue their existence.

On March 6, 2012, in Sunnyvale, California, Elizabeth Hodgins shot and killed her 22-year-old son, George, and then committed suicide. George was autistic. Zoe Gross reports:

> [Commentators] said that they felt sympathy for the mother. They called her George's "guardian angel." They said no one should judge her unless they had walked in her shoes. They said that it wasn't wrong because he was autistic, and autistic children are hell to raise. They said that it wasn't wrong because she was obviously responding to a lack of services. (In fact, she had refused services.) They said that it wasn't wrong because he was disabled, and so his life couldn't have been very good anyway. (2012)

Two days later, Canadian Robert Latimer responded to George's murder with a television appearance. In 1993, Latimer murdered his 12-year-old daughter Tracy, who had cerebral palsy. Latimer trapped Tracy in his truck and exposed her to carbon monoxide gas. According to Gross:

> Robert Latimer went on television to talk about how loving and compassionate it was when he gassed his disabled daughter Tracy. He called for "euthanasia"—the murder of disabled children by their parents—to be legalized in Canada. A woman who appeared with him agreed. She has two disabled children who she would like to kill, but she can't because it is against the law. No opposing viewpoints were presented. (2012)

In 2010, 17-year-old Leosha Barnett died of malnutrition in Fort Worth, Texas. Reportedly, Leosha was cognitively limited and had epilepsy, but was not receiving medical care at the time of her death. Leosha was starved to death by her mother, Tasca Kuniko Stevenson, and her sister, Kyreshi Stevenson. Tasca Stevenson's lawyer commented after arrests were made:

> This child was not expected to live from birth. She had a myriad of medical problems, but she lived until she was 17. Kyreshi's mother was going through some personal issues. [Stevenson] was trying to take care of her kid and her mother's children, and I think she was overwhelmed by everything, but nothing was done intentionally. (Fort Worth Star-Telegram 2010)

On this interpretation of her murder, Leosha's life becomes the anomalous event while her death is treated as a matter of course. When she was killed, 5-foot 4-inch Leosha weighed only 79.8 pounds. Leosha's mother visited the house where Leosha lived with her sister frequently (2–3 times per week). Yet, at the time of her death, Stevenson testified that she had not seen her daughter for four months. Leosha was being held in her room.

In 2013, 14-year-old Alex Spourdalakis was murdered in River Grove, Illinois. "After failing to kill him with sleeping pills, [his mother and godmother] stabbed him in the chest repeatedly before slitting his wrists" ("ASAN calls" 2013). Alex was murdered because he was autistic; the murder was premeditated (*ibid.*). According to the Autism Self Advocacy Network:

> Many in the media have attempted to excuse Alex's murder or sympathize with his killers, citing the challenges of his disability and the need to improve the quality and availability of service-provision . . . His death is not about services, nor is it about the difficulties associated with his disability. Prior to murdering him, Alex's mother was offered and refused services from the Illinois Department of Children and Family Services. In truth, Alex's murder is about a reprehensible and repulsive ideology all too common within our society that preaches that it is better to be dead than disabled. *As long as our society treats the lives of disabled people as worth less than those of the general population, more disabled children and adults will be subject to acts of violence and murder.* (2013, emphasis mine)

Like Spourdalakis, Barnett, Hodgins, and Latimer, Daniel Corby was murdered because he was disabled. The 4-year-old autistic child was drowned in a bathtub by his mother, Patricia, in San Diego, California in the spring of 2012. According to the prosecutor on the case, "[Patricia] told police that the boy was autistic and that she didn't believe he would have a life or a future without her, so she decided to kill him" (Littlefield 2012).

Beliefs held by the parents and commentators I highlight above are continuous with beliefs expressed in mainstream bioethics literature, which repeatedly assumes that the lives of persons with disabilities are less valuable. Bioethicist Sara Goering analyzes instances in which bioethicists reject the testimony of persons with disabilities who insist their quality of life is high. She categorizes these responses into two groups, which she calls "accusation of denial"—when bioethicists assume that individuals in question are in denial about their unhappiness and would take a magic pill to cure their disability if it was available—and "accusation of lowered expectations" which maps onto adaptive preference literature in feminist theory (2008, 126). Goering's interpretation of these dismissive claims is intuitively correct: they imply there is a way to objectively rank the quality of lives and bodies. This is precisely the ableist ideology that the Autism Advocacy Network says is "responsible" for these murders, and it is one that also conditions bioethics literature and the thinking of radical enhancement enthusiasts.

RATIONING

The murder cases in the previous section are infuriatingly continuous with the treatment of persons with disabilities globally. People with disabilities are impoverished, abused, neglected, raped, and cut off from the economy, politics, and family life. When we talk about disability rights, we are talking about already-existing persons, and the social and political goods which fluctuate in an inverse relationship to the construction of a justifiably rejectable other (cf. Saxton 2000, 158). Ableism can curb or eliminate the distribution of social and political goods (like appropriate housing, medical insurance, transportation, and other goods and necessities) to perceived members of disability communities.[4] This problem implicates and flows into the medical realm, where persons with disabilities are especially vulnerable and regularly experience the barriers of marginalization and prejudice.

The actuarial thinking I discussed in Chapter 4 and continue to discuss here is amplified through practices and discourses of medical resource rationing. Stigma against persons with disabilities related to genetic counseling should be framed within the context of the increased mainstream certainty, especially in the United States, that rationing health care is necessary, and because of various proposed means by which this rationing would be carried out (e.g. Fleck 2009). The technical meaning of "quality of life," along with its measure, QALYs (Quality-Adjusted Life Years), was developed in the context of rationing and questions regarding the efficiency of health care. These quantitative concepts have nothing to do with subjective satisfaction; they are deployed to measure health-care efficacy. A system of objective measures estimating quality of life calls into question, especially, the provision of expensive health-care measures to ill, disabled, and elderly persons

(Amundson 2006). As aforementioned, Savulescu has explicitly called into question the appeal of equality of access when he considers cardiac care for persons with Down syndrome (2001c). Meanwhile, a recent "secret shopper" style study shows that persons using wheelchairs are already denied access to subspecialty medical care (gynecology and psychiatry, among others), although no strong rationing procedures currently exist (Lagu *et al.* 2013). This is true despite the legal provisions of the Americans with Disabilities Act meant to protect equal access. The study found:

> Of 256 practices, 56 (22%) reported that they could not accommodate the patient, 9 (4%) reported that the building was inaccessible, 47 (18%) reported inability to transfer a patient from a wheelchair to an examination table, and 22 (9%) reported use of height-adjustable tables or a lift for transfer. Gynecology was the subspecialty with the highest rate of inaccessible practices (44%). (Lagu *et al.* 2013, 441)

Today's rationing conversations occur in an environment which already excludes and therefore stigmatizes persons with disabilities.

With regard to genetic enhancement and selection, bald cost-benefit analyzes are often made. For instance, bioethicist Daniel Brock, in a talk regarding the prevention of "severe disabilities," argued that "it's a mistake to think that the social and economic costs are not a legitimate concern in this context" (quoted in Tremain 2006, n. 3). Genetic screening for Fragile-X was undertaken in the 1990s under explicitly economic terms. Proponents in Colorado noted that "the savings for the state" resulting from testing and selective abortion would be "tremendous" compared to the cost of caring for those with cognitive impairment connected to the presence of Fragile-X (Nelson and Lindee 1995, 162–163). In 1989, an insurance company refused to cover the child resulting from a fetus which tested positively for cystic fibrosis, citing the fact that the child would have a pre-existing condition (Thompson 1989). Happily, GINA, the Genetic Information Nondiscrimination Act of 2008, "prohibits discrimination by health insurers and employers on the basis of genetic information" (*InteliHealth* 2014). But, such laws are not consistent with the goals and aims of transhumanist futures.

The certainty of particular conditions and related characteristics for potential children varies according to what condition one considers and the specific tests and screening procedures applied. A nuanced look at these issues is undercut by the influence of genetic determinism which undergirds the cost-benefit analysis and rationing philosophy that drives and motivates testing and screening in public policy arenas. Genetic information must be taken very seriously as compared to environmental, behavioral, and other factors in order for the conclusions of such cost-benefit analyzes to make sense. One must be reasonably certain that costs will decrease as a result of testing and selection and must downplay the costs of health care for "unmarked" fetuses (those that pass testing and selection procedures). This type of actuarial thinking is highly suspect and, as I have argued, is structured by the idea that chance is a biological matter that can be rooted out. Its everyday usage and acceptability structures disability in particular as a risk (of pregnancy, of genetic deviance) and so persons with disabilities become the inhabitants of risky and preventable bodies, the blame for which lies outside of social and political institutions.

CONCLUSION

Disability rights projects and advocacy should tackle the issues covered in this chapter, and transhumanism presents no resources to do so; in fact, transhumanist thinking provides theoretical support for linking disability with risk. My consideration of the transhumanist strategies of transcending embodiment and selecting embryos in earlier chapters of this book yields the conclusion that transhumanism does not ameliorate stigmas connected with disability. Instead, transhumanism can exacerbate ableism. Transhumanists strategies aim to create bulwarks against risk—risks associated with embodied vulnerability and genetic deviance. The portrait of embodiment as risk in transhumanist accounts establishes disability as the symbol of a feared outcome and a stand-in for death. Instead of seeing disability as a complex interrelationship between the body, social structures, and social norms, disability is reduced to a biological fact about the body and reframed as the outcome of technophobia and a too-complacent posture toward death.

Transhumanists seek to eliminate or mitigate dependence and vulnerability, while disability rights proponents seek to drain stigmatizing power from these concepts and embrace differences of all kinds. Transhumanists make a universalizing gesture when they categorize all humans as deficient, but this move serves to merely shift, rather than ameliorate, stigma connected to deficiency—thus maintaining and even strengthening ableism. Transhumanists enjoy strong institutional influence in bioethics and have advanced arguments in regard to which particular human traits are required for a life of quality. In effect, they ask the biopolitical question: Who should live? Ensuing discussions affect all people whose lives are taken to be inherently less valuable than the lives of other people, but they especially affect the lives of persons with disabilities. We must fight ableism, in all its forms—from the genetic counselor's office to the family home—if we are to fight the violence and neglect to which persons with disabilities are too often subject.

NOTES

1. Since its launch, the company was issued a warning letter from the Food and Drug Administration, which objected to its issue of 200 reports and ancestry information on the basis of DNA testing on saliva. Because 23andMe was issue what appeared to be diagnoses, the FDA claims that it is subject to its approval. Attempting to comply, 23andMe has begun to submit its health reports to the FDA for approval (Hof 2014).

2. But testing can be undertaken on *behalf* of the fetus. For example, in the case of fetal diagnosis of PKU (phenylketonuria), dietary changes alone can almost erase the impact that this metabolic disorder can have on bodily function. These dietary changes cannot be made unless doctors and parents are aware of the diagnosis. A second example is Rh negative disease, which refers to the conditions in the womb when the mother has a negative blood type and the fetus has a positive blood type. The mother's body has an auto-immune reaction to the fetus's blood and begins to destroy the fetus's red blood cells (Gale 2012). Lacking this information gleaned through amniocentesis, the condition is fatal immediately after birth.

3. For more on the topic of risk, pregnancy and biopolitics from feminist perspectives see the work of Catherine Mills (2011) and Lorna Weir (1996, 2006).

4. It is important to recall, as James Charlton points out, that individuals do not usually choose whether or not they are disabled—that choice is made for them (Riley 2005, 8–9).

Conclusion

Rethinking the Future

While transhumanists proclaim that futuristic technology opens the door to greater diversity in the human form and capability, transhumanist enhancement strategies—which perpetuate the power of deviance as a normative concept—belie that aim. Opening up the future to diverse forms of life would require the mitigation of the stigma of disability, which in turn would require revisiting the terms upon which ideals of normality are constructed. Instead, transhumanists operate with a thick sense of what counts as normal and recommend strategies for enhancement which are largely synonymous with refusing to create persons with disabilities, a eugenic goal directly in opposition to the goals of disability rights. The goals of transhumanism and disability rights are not only disparate, but are in the most important respect fundamentally opposed; transhumanist futures exclude disability, while disabled futures are expansive and inclusive.

In a striking analysis of novelist Marge Piercy's *Woman on the Edge of Time* (1976), feminist philosopher of disability Alison Kafer argues that for Piercy, and many feminists reading the novel, it makes sense that the feminist future of this science fiction fantasy does not include persons with disabilities—most do not call this feature into question (2011). In fact, the reproductive technology which makes gender parity possible in the novel also is imagined to preclude the existence of persons with disabilities. Piercy's hoped-for participatory democracy is demonstrated in the novel by way of a debate among its characters; this debate is over whether the reproductive technology should be used to merely eliminate "genes linked to birth defects and disease susceptibility" or to "select for 'positive' traits" (220). Kafer writes: "It is taken for granted by both sides—and by Piercy and (presumably) her audience—that everyone knows and agrees which genes and characteristics are negative and therefore which ones should be eliminated; questions about so-called negative traits are apparently not worth discussing" (221).

Kafer extends her analysis to discuss the story of Sharon Duchesneau and Candace McCullough, the deaf lesbians discussed in Chapter 4 who use a deaf sperm donor and met fierce opposition in the media (223). Kafer suggests that we need counter narratives, stories like Duchesneau and McCullough's, to balance the ideology of the cure: "'curing' and eliminating disability—whether through stem cell research or selective abortion—is almost always presented as a universally valued goal about which there can, and should, be no disagreement" (2011, 236; cf. e.g. Harris 2011, 147). We need stories like "people embracing their bodies, proudly proclaiming disability as sexy, powerful, and worthy; tales of disabled parents and parents with disabled children refusing to accept that a bright future . . . precludes disability and asserting the right to bear and keep children with disabilities . . ." (237). Kafer notes that these stories are contested and can be inconsistent, but that they "deserve telling" (237).

Internationally known transhumanists like Nick Bostrom, James Hughes, and Julian Savulescu share a basic premise: human beings have strong moral obligations to enhance themselves and their children. Transhumanists identify untapped potential in evolving technologies, including genetics, robotics, informatics, nanotechnology (GRIN) and related fields to wholly revolutionize the human being and, transhumanists claim, thereby create a better world (Garreau 2005 and Rubin 2008). Transhumanists seek to usher in an improved future by paving the way for posthumanity, the presumed result of enhancing today's human beings who will, eventually, be radically overcome. These thinkers believe prejudices regarding the boundaries or sanctity of human nature and status quo bias present formidable roadblocks on the path to a posthuman, utopian future (Hughes 2007). Academic transhumanists and popular writers like Ray Kurzweil are joined in their call for radical enhancement by some bioethicists, including John Harris and Jonathan Glover. Harris and Glover also claim that enhancing individuals will improve society as a whole; although they do not call themselves "transhumanists," they can nevertheless be referred to as "enhancement enthusiasts" and "fellow travelers" in the transhumanist project (Koch 2010).

In this book, I challenged these views and argued that transhumanists implicitly and explicitly question the existence and value of persons in the disability community. I traced the borders of the social acceptance of particular bodies and iterations of the bio political question: who should live? I investigated the fantasies of transhumanism and exposed the ableist assumptions and heritage which drive and shape it. My motivation, here, was to track the denigration of dependence, difference, and the body, alongside the overvaluation of the avoidance of death, longevity, and intelligence (of a particular kind) in bioethics literature. My main focusing question was: what desires or wishes do transhumanist utopias represent, and what can these utopias teach us about ableism in bioethical contexts? I found that transhumanist strategies reinscribe disability onto the body, ignoring its social contours and construction.

As exemplified in the work of Bostrom and Savulescu, transhumanism views the current human body through the lens of risk, and views biotechnology through the lens of choice. The risk that the human body encounters is often conceived of as the risk of disablement, including disablement through aging, illness or accident. For these thinkers, then, and we who are under the same spell, the disabled body is uniquely linked in a false chain of equivalences to limitation, risk, and death. In contrast to this body, transhumanist utopias focus on an ideal subject, one which would experience no restriction with regard to pleasures, choice-making, or opportunities—the techno-liberal subject, a subject whose future is mediated by the choice to use technology. This fixation on a utopian version of what the human subject should be comes at the expense of already-existing persons.

In carrying out my research, I was committed to understanding disability in such a way that would recognize the centrality of society's responsibility to make a place for, respond to, and attend to persons and their needs. I carried out my attempt by revisiting the terms of philosophical debate in bioethics, the provision of medical care, political institutions, and institutional barriers of all kinds. I was also committed to using Foucault's framework of biopolitics as a jumping-off point to engage the special points of contact between enhancement enthusiasm and disability. Each section of the preceding pages represents an engagement with the ways in which meanings and definitions of disability are built and sustained in various social, political, and philosophical contexts—that is, a variety of "locations" of disability were explored.

In Chapter 1, I discussed bioethics literature on enhancement and introduced transhumanist thinking, demonstrating that transhumanist visions impact and are impacted by bioethics literature more generally. In Chapter 2, I discussed disability within a variety of political contexts, both practical and theoretical, and laid out an understanding of disability as a floating cultural concept layered upon stigma and deviance. In Chapter 3, I investigated a history of enhancement technologies, which is also a history of how illness and deviance, and therefore disability, have been defined against changing conceptions of health. In Chapter 4, in many ways the heart of the book, I called into question the implicit naturalization of disability inherent in Julian Savulescu's suggestion that negative genetic selection is not only a desirable "human enhancement" technique but also a moral obligation. There, I also discussed disability in the context of disability rights and critically evaluated the potential of transhumanist thinking to contribute to disability rights projects. Throughout the chapter, I attempted to delineate and work from a position which seeks reproductive justice and is pointedly critical of the deeply ableist context in which prenatal testing technology is developed, employed, and recommended by the medical community to women and parent(s) who are expecting. In Chapter 5, I investigated genetic counseling practices, the identification of disability with risk, and the ways ableist discourses place persons with disabilities at risk.

For the transhumanist, positive and negative eugenics are linked together. While these "strategies" of enhancement are often tackled as separate, I have argued that there are theoretical and practical connections between these two strategies and that transhumanists cannot help but implicitly acknowledge their connection. Transhumanism treats the two modes as co-extensive: to rid the world of disability *is* to enhance the human. Recall that Savulescu claims that we must enhance or go extinct, and that his preferred mode of enhancement is genetic selection (selection against marked embryos). Transhumanism here enacts a reversal of the feminist insight that subjectivity is interconnected and persons are significantly interdependent; transhumanists perversely acknowledge the importance of intersubjectivity when they implicitly claim that for the population to be enhanced, deviance must be eilminated. This is the heart of the linkage between positive and negative eugenics and the biopolitical logic I have attempted to draw out in these pages—enhancement seems to require, for the transhumanist, the rejection of disability and embodiment generally as risk and limitation. This rejection is posed as necessary for the realization of enhancement for the individual and even in order to save the world (Savulescu 2009).

In many ways, transhumanism is an expression of its setting in bioethics, and bioethics is in turn influenced by transhumanism. In this theoretical milieu, one gets the impression that reproduction would be perfected if women were not involved at all—the womb is a risky place for the fetus to gestate. In an echo of the all-too-familiar duality at the center of Enlightenment's humanism, women represent chance and we are urged to take up the rationality necessary to counter this issue; as Niccolò Machiavelli infamously put it, ". . . fortune is a woman, and it is necessary, if you wish to master her, to conquer her by force" (1950, 94). Transhumanist argumentation transforms all embodiment into risk—recall Bostrom's imagery of the paper hut, and Savulescu's treatment of reproduction as a risky game of Wheel of Fortune. Against this backdrop, the fetus becomes a special site of risk—especially the risk of disability—and autonomous "reproducers" should embrace their role as risk managers in order to stave off undesirable outcomes.

Transhumanism sees freedom as the freedom to make choices, and the freedom to make choices as positioned as a route to bliss and happiness. Transhumanism extends the prerogatives of humanism instead of calling its boundaries into question. Transhumanism seeks a broader field of action, proliferating choices, a secure future—not transgressed boundaries and transformative hybridity. In many ways, transhumanism disappoints the radical. Transhumanist enhancement is simply a romantic dream of endless autonomy. "Better" and "best" for the transhumanist references social prejudices without questioning them. Finally, the "freedom" of choice-making is opposed to the "risks" of disability and embodiment; transhumanism reinforces boundary lines between disability and ability. Because transhumanist visions of the future do not question stigmas, these visions serve to reify them.

In conclusion, I offer a suggestion for further philosophical reflection on the future and political action on the issues brought up in the course of this project. A revised version of *enhanced futures* could focus on the revision of political and social circumstances, seeking justice for those with disabilities and acceptance of diverse forms of embodiment. Enhancement strategies, and the reasoning behind them, should be critically examined. But, this critical examination always gestures toward truly transformative, critical enhancement strategies. Cost-and-benefit analyses connected to the bio political question of who should live must be challenged. We should seek reproductive justice that begins to take apart discourses of sexism and ableism and reject the so-called reproductive liberty offered through participation in the industries of reproductive technologies. Appropriate housing, transportation, schooling, and medical care must be sought. These would be true "enhancements" that would bring about better futures. Enhancement can be made an expression of care, care of existing individuals—not idealized future subjects that cannot, and will not, exist.

We should *seek* augmentations—political, social, and technological—that bridge the gap between the body and individual life goals as articulated by those upon whom the suggested technology would intervene; this makes enhancement an expression of care and interdependence, and would resemble neither positive nor negative eugenics. We should *reject* enhancement strategies which rely, for their desirability, on ableist discourses of risk which fetishize autonomy and choice and visions of happiness that depend on added capabilities rather than complex interdependence.

Bibliography

23andMe. 2013. Accessed April 14. https://www.23andme.com/.

Abberley, Paul. 1987. "The Concept of Oppression and the Development of a Social Theory of Disability." *Disability, Handicap and Society* 21: 5–19.

Adams, Mark. 2009. *Mr. America: How Muscular Millionaire Bernarr Macfadden Transformed the Nation Through Sex, Salad, and the Ultimate Starvation Diet.* HarperCollins.

Agar, Nicholas. 2004. *Liberal Eugenics: In Defence of Human Enhancement.* Oxford: Blackwell Publishing.

———. 2007. "Whereto Transhumanism? The Literature Reaches a Critical Mass." *Hastings Center Report* 37, No. 3: 12–17.

———. 2010. *Humanity's End: Why We Should Reject Radical Enhancement.* Cambridge: The MIT Press.

———. 2013. *Truly Human Enhancement: A Philosophical Defense of Limits.* Cambridge: The MIT Press.

Aiken, Scott, and Robert Talisse. 2014. *Why We Argue (And How We Should): A Guide to Political Disagreement.* New York: Routledge.

Amundson, Ron. 2000. "Against Normal Function." *Studies in History, Philosophy, Biology and Biomedical Science* 31, No. 1: 33–53.

———. 2006. "Health Resource Rationing." In *Encyclopedia of Disability* Vol. 2, edited by Gary Albrecht, 841–845. Sage Publications.

Are You Fit to Marry? 1927. Film. John E. Allen, Inc. [first released as *The Black Stork*, 1917]."ASAN calls for Federal Hate Crime Prosecution for the Murder of Alex Spourdalakis." 2013.

Autistic Self Advocacy Network, June 18. Accessed June 15, 2014: htttp://www.autisticadvocacy.org.

Asch, Adrienne. 1989. "Reproductive Technology and Disability." In *Reproductive Laws for the 1990's*, edited by Sherrill Cohen and Nadine Taub, 69–124. Clifton, NJ: Humana Press.

———. 2000a. "Comments on Severe Impairment and the Beginning of Life." *APA Newsletter on Philosophy and Medicine* 99, No. 2 (Spring).

———. 2000b. "Why I Haven't Changed My Mind About Prenatal Diagnosis: Reflections and Refinements." In *Prenatal Testing and Disability Rights*, edited by Erik Parens and Adrienne Asch. Washington, DC: Georgetown University Press.

———. 2003. "Disability Equality and Prenatal Testing: Contradictory or Compatible?" *Florida State University Law Review* 30: 315.

———. 2006. "Appearance-Altering Surgery: Children's Sense of Self, and Parental Love." In *Surgically Shaping Children: Technology, Ethics, and the Pursuit of Normality*, edited by Erik Parens, 227–252. Baltimore: Johns Hopkins University Press.

Asch, Adrienne and Gail Gellner. 1996. "Feminism, Bioethics and Genetics." In *Feminism and Bioethics*, edited by Susan M. Wolf, 318–350. New York: Oxford University Press.

Asch, Adrienne and David T. Wasserman. 2005. "Where's the Sin in Synecdoche?" In *Quality of Life and Human Difference: Genetic Testing, Health Care, and Disability*, edited by David T. Wasserman, Robert Samuel Wachbroit, and Jerome Edmund Bickenbach, 172–216. New York: Cambridge University Press.

"Asperger's Syndrome Dropped from Psychiatrists' Handbook the DSM." 2012. *The Guardian*, Dec 12. Accessed March 26, 2013. http://www.guardian.co.uk/society/2012/dec/02/aspergers-syndrome-dropped-psychiatric-dsm.

Aspinall, Cassandra. 2006. "Do I Make You Uncomfortable? Reflections on Using Surgery to Reduce the Distress of Others." In *Surgically Shaping Children: Technology, Ethics, and the Pursuit of Normality*, edited by Erik Parens, 13–28. Baltimore: Johns Hopkins University Press.

Baillie, Harold and Casey, Timothy, eds. 2005. *Is Human Nature Obsolete? Genetics, Bioengineering and the Future of the Human Condition.* Cambridge, MA: The MIT Press.

Baltimore, David, Paul Berg, Michael Botchan, Dana Carroll, R. Alta Charo, George Church, Jacob E. Corn, George Q. Daley, Jennifer A. Doudna, Marsha Fenner, Henry T. Greely, Martin Jinek, G. Steven Martin, Edward Penhoet, Jennifer Puck, Samuel H. Sternberg, Jonathan S. Weissman, and Keith R. Yamamoto. 2015. "A Prudent Path Forward for Genomic Engineering and Germline Gene Modification." *Science* 348, No. 6230: 36–38.

Bartky, Sandra. 2005. "On psychological oppression." In *Feminist theory: A philosophical anthology*, edited by Ann E. Cudd and Robin O. Andreasen, 105–114. Massachusetts: Blackwell Publishing.

Battleday, Ruairidh M. and Anna-Katharine Brem. 2015. "Modafinil for Cognitive Neuroenhancement in Healthy Non-Sleep-Deprived Subjects: A Systematic Review." *European Neuropsychopharmacology* 25: 1865–1881.

Bauman, Zygmunt. 1989. *Modernity and the Holocaust*. Ithaca, NY: Cornell University Press.

Begley, Sharon. 2015. "Medical First: Gene-Editing Tool used to Treat Girl's Cancer." *STAT: Reporting from the frontiers of health and medicine*, November 5. Accessed July 30, 2016. https://www.statnews.com/2015/11/05/doctors-report-first-use-gene-editing-technology-patient/.

Bennett, Jim. 2012. "Weakness—a Crime!" Accessed April 28. www.bernarrmacfadden.com/macfadden3.html

Bernasconi, Robert. 2010. "The Policing of Race Mixing: The Place of Biopower within the History of Racisms." *Bioethical Inquiry* 7: 205–216.

Bostrom, Nick. 2004. "The Future of Human Evolution." Accessed July 31, 2016. www.nickbostrom.com/fut/evolution.html.

———. 2005a. "The Fable of the Dragon-Tyrant." *Journal of Medical Ethics* 31, No. 5: 273–277.

———. 2005b. "In Defense of Posthuman Dignity." *Bioethics* 19: 202–214.

———. 2005c. "A History of Transhumanist Thought." *Journal of Evolution and Technology* 14, No. 1: 1–25.

———. 2005d. "Humanity's Biggest Problems Aren't What You Think They Are." *TED*. Accessed December 1, 2012. http://www.youtube.com/watch?v=Yd9cf_vLviI.

———. 2008. "Why I Want to Be a Posthuman When I Grow Up." In *Medical Enhancement and Humanity*, edited by Bert Gordijn and Ruth Chadwick, 107–136. Springer.

———. 2009. "Transhumanist Values." In *Contemporary Bioethics: A Reader with Cases,* edited by Jessica Pierce and George Randels, 619–624. Originally published in *Journal of Philosophical Research* 30 (Supplement): 3–14.

———. 2010. "Letter from Utopia." Accessed June 15, 2012. www.nickbostrom.com/utopia.

———. 2012. "Human Genetic Enhancements: A Transhumanist Perspective." In *Arguing About Bioethics,* edited by Stephen Holland, 105–114. Originally published in *Journal of Value Inquiry* 37, No. 4: 493–506.

Bostrom, Nick and Toby Ord. 2006. "The Reversal Test: Eliminating Status Quo Bias in Applied Ethics." *Ethics* 116, No. 4: 656–679.

Bostrom, Nick and Anders Sandberg. 2011. "The Wisdom of Nature: An Evolutionary Heuristic for Human Enhancement." In *Human Enhancement*, edited by Julian Savulescu and Nick Bostrom, 375–416. Oxford, UK: Oxford University Press.

Bostrom, Nick and Julian Savulescu. 2011. "Human Enhancement Ethics: The State of the Debate." In *Human Enhancement*, edited by Julian Savulescu and Nick Bostrom, 1–22. Oxford, UK: Oxford University Press.

Boyle, Robert J. and Julian Savulescu. 2003. "Prenatal Diagnosis for 'Minor' Genetic Abnormalities is Ethical." *The American Journal of Bioethics* 3, No. 1 (Winter): 60–65.

Brave, Ralph. 2003. "James Watson Wants to Build a Better Human." *AlterNet*, May 29. Accessed April 6, 2013. http://www.alternet.org/story/16026/james_watson_wants_to_build_a_better_human.

Brock, Daniel. 1992. "The Human Genome Project and Human Identity." *Houston Law Review* 29, No. 1: 7–22.

———. 1998. "Enhancements of Human Function: Some Distinctions for Policymakers." In *Enhancing Human Traits*, edited by Erik Parens: 48–69.

———. 2009. "Is Selection of Children Wrong?" In *Human Enhancement*, edited by Julian Savulescu and Nick Bostrom. Oxford: Oxford University Press.

Brownlee, Kimberley and Adam Cureton, eds. 2009. *Disability and Disadvantage*. Oxford: Oxford University Press.

Buchanan, Allen. 2011a. *Better Than Human: The Promise and Perils of Enhancing Ourselves*. Oxford: Oxford University Press.

———. 2011b. *Beyond Humanity?* Oxford: Oxford University Press.

Buchanan, Allen, Daniel Brock, Norman Daniels and Daniel Wikler. 2000. *From Chance to Choice: Genetics and Justice*. Cambridge: Cambridge University Press.

Buck, Claudia. 2016. "Deaf People Encounter Troubles with Medical Care." *The Sacramento Bee* July 11. Accessed July 26, 2016. http://www.sacbee.com/news/local/health-and-medicine/article88784482.html.

Brueggemann, Brenda Jo, Linda Feldmeier White, Patricia A. Dunn, Barbara A. Heifferon and Johnson Cheu. 2001. "Becoming Visible: Lessons in Disability." *College Composition and Communication* 52, No. 3 (February): 368–398.

Byrd, W. Carson, and Matthew W. Hughey. 2015. "Born that Way? 'Scientific' Racism is Creeping Back into Our Thinking. Here's What to Watch Out For." *WashingtonPost.com*, September 28. Accessed July 26, 2016.https://www.washingtonpost.com/blogs/monkey-cage/wp/2015/09/28/born-that-way-scientific-racism-is-creeping-back-into-our-thinking-heres-what-to-watch-out-for/

Carlson, Licia. 2002. "The Morality of Prenatal Testing and Selective Abortion: Clarifying the Expressivist Objection." In *Mutating Concepts, Evolving Disciplines: Genetics, Medicine and Society*, edited by L. S. Parker and R. A. Ankeny, 191–213. Netherlands: Kluwer Academic Publishers.

———. 2009. *The Faces of Intellectual Disability: Philosophical Reflections*. Indianapolis: Indiana University Press.

Charlton, James L. 1998. *Nothing About Us Without Us: Disability Oppression and Empowerment*. Berkeley: University of California Press.

———. 2010. "The Dimensions of Disability Oppression." In *The Disability Studies Reader*, edited by Lennard J. Davis, 147–159. New York: Routledge.

Chandler, E., Gill, Henry M., Taylor, K. T. Lin, Bimal B. Padaliya, William J. Newman, Anna I. Abramovitch, CaraLee R. Richardson, P. David Charles. 2006. "Difficulty in Securing Treatment for Degenerative Hip Disease in a Patient with Down Syndrome: The Gap Remains Open." *Journal of the National Medical Association* 98, No. 1 (January): 93–96.

Clare, Eli. 1999. *Exile and Pride: Disability, Queerness and Liberation*. Cambridge: South End Press.

Coady, A.J. 2011. "Playing God." In *Human Enhancement*, edited by Julian Savulescu and Nick Bostrom, 155–180. Oxford: Oxford University Press.

Cohen, Elizabeth. 2013. "Disabled Baby Denied Heart Transplant." *CNN.com*, November 30. Accessed July 26, 2016. http://www.cnn.com/2013/11/30/health/disabled-transplants/.

Coleman Brown, Lerita M. 2010. "Stigma: An Enigma Demystified." In *The Disability Studies Reader*, edited by Lennard J. Davis, 179–192. New York: Routledge.

Conrad, Peter. 1997. "Public Eyes and Private Genes: Historical Frames, News, Constructions, and Social Problems." *Social Problems* 44: 139–154.

———. 2002. "Genetics and Behavior in the News: Dilemmas of a Rising Paradigm." In *The Double-Edged Helix: Social Implications of Genetics in a Diverse Society*, edited by J. S. Alper, C. Ard, A. Asch, J. Beckwith, P. Conrad, & L. N. Geller, 58–79. Baltimore, MD: Johns Hopkins University Press.

Crook, Paul. 2008. "The New Eugenics? The Ethics of Bio-Technology." *Australian Journal of Politics and History* 54, No. 1 (March): 135–143.

Daniels, Norman. 1985. *Just Health Care*. Princeton, NJ: Princeton University Press.

———. 2011. "Can Anyone Really Be Talking About Ethically Modifying Human Nature?" In *Human Enhancement*, edited by Julian Savulescu and Nick Bostrom, 25–42. Oxford, UK: Oxford University Press.

Daniels, Norman, Susannah Rose, and Ellen Zide (2009). "Disability, Adaptation, and Inclusion." In *Disability and Disadvantage*, edited by Kimberley Brownlee and Adam Cureton, 54–85. Oxford: Oxford University Press.

Dar-Nimrod, Ilan, and Steven J. Heine. 2010. "Genetic Essentialism: On the Deceptive Determinism of DNA." *Psychological Bulletin* December 13 (Advance online publication). doi: 10.1037/a0021860.

Davis, Dena. 1997. "Genetic Dilemmas and the Child's Right to an Open Future." *The Hastings Center Report* 27, No. 2 (March–April): 7–15.

———. 2010. *Genetic Dilemmas: Reproductive Technology, Parental Choices, and Children's Futures*. Oxford: Oxford University Press.

Davis, Lennard J. 2002. "Bodies of Difference: Politics, Disability, and Representation." In *Disability Studies: Enabling the Humanities*, edited by Brenda Jo Brueggemann, Sharon L. Snyder, and Rosemarie Garland-Thomson, 101–106. New York: Modern Language Association.

de Melo-Martín, Immaculada. 2005. "Firing Up the Nature/Nurture Controversy: Bioethics and Genetic Determinism." *J Med Ethics* 31: 526–530.

Dell Orto, Arthur E. and Robert P. Marinelli, eds. 1995. *Encyclopedia of Disability and Rehabilitation*. Macmillan Library Reference USA.

Dennett, Daniel. 2013. *Intuition Pumps and Other Tools for Thinking*. New York: W.W. Norton & Company.

Derrida, Jacques. 2005. *Rogues: Two Essays on Reason*. Translated by Pascale-Anne Brault and Michael Naas. Palo Alto: Stanford University Press.

Dhanda, Rahul K. 2002. *Guiding Icarus: Merging Bioethics with Corporate Interests*. John Wiley & Sons.

Diament, Michelle. 2012a. "Sheltered Workshops Offer Little Benefit, Studies Find." *Disability Scoop* February 21. Accessed September 4.http://www.disabilityscoop.com/2012/02/21/sheltered-workshops-benefit/15035.

———. 2012b. "Most Federal Dollars Go to Sheltered Workshops." *Disability Scoop* April 4. Accessed September 4. http://www.disabilityscoop.com/2012/04/04/most-dollars-workshops/15318.

———. 2013. "Doctors Turning Away Patients with Disabilities." *Disability Scoop* March 19. Accessed March 19.www.disabilityscoop.com/2013/03/19/doctors-turning-away/17518/print/.

Dvorsky, George. 2003. "And the Disabled Shall Inherit the Earth." *Sentient Developments: Science, Futurism, Life*. September 13, 2003.

Elliott, Carl. 2004. *Better than Well: American Medicine Meets the American Dream*. New York: W. W. Norton & Company.

———. 2011. "Enhancement Technologies and the Modern Self." *Journal of Medicine and Philosophy* 36: 364–374.

Ellis, Kathleen. 2003. “Reinforcing the Stigma: The Representation of Disability in Gattaca.” *Australian Screen Education Online* 31: 111–114.

———. 2007. “Disability as Visual Shorthand: Theme and Style in Australian Cinema in the 1990s.” *Metro* 152 (Autumn): 135–139.

Engelhardt, H. Tristram. 1984. “Persons and Humans: Re-Fashioning Ourselves in a Better Image and Likeness.” *Zygon* 19: 281–295.

———. 1990. “Human Nature Technologically Revisited.” *Social Philosophy and Policy* 8: 180–191.

Engster, Daniel. 2005. “Rethinking Care Theory: The Practice of Caring and the Obligation to Care.” *Hypatia* 20, No. 3: 50–74.

Entman, Robert and Andrew Rojecky. 2001. *The Black Image in the White Mind: Media and Race in America*. Chicago: University of Chicago Press.

Ernst, Robert. 1991. *Weakness Is a Crime: The Life of Bernarr Mcfadden*. New York: Syracuse University Press.

Ervin, Mike. 2009. “Jerry Lewis Doesn’t Deserve a Humanitarian Award at the Oscars.” *The Progressive*. Accessed April 6, 2013. http://www.progressive.org/mag/mplewis021909.html.

Fair, John D. 2012. “Physical Culture.” *Encyclopedia Britannica*. Accessed April 9.https://www.britannica.com/topic/physical-culture.

Feinberg, Joel. 1980. “The Child’s Right to an Open Future.” In *Whose Child? Children’s Rights, Parental Authority, and State Power*, edited by William Aiken and Hugh LaFollette, 124–153. Totowa, NJ: Rowman & Littlefield.

Fine, Michael. 2005. “Dependency Work: A Critical Exploration of Kittay’s Perspective on Care as a Relationship of Power.” *Health Sociology Review* 14, No. 2: 146–160.

Fineman, Martha L. 2002. “Masking Dependency: The Political Role of Family Rhetoric.” In *The Subject of Care: Feminist Perspectives on Dependency,* edited by Eva Feder Kittay and Ellen K. Feder, 215–244. New York: Rowman & Littlefield.

Finger, Anna. 2007. “What Is It with All the Napkins?” *Disability Studies Quarterly* 27, No. 3.

Firestone, Shulamith. 1970. *The Dialectic of Sex: The Case for Feminist Revolution*. New York: Bantam Books.

Fisher, Irving and Eugene Fisk. 1916. *How to Live: Rules for Healthful Living Based on Modern Science*. Funk & Wagnalls Company.

Fitzgerald, Kelly. 2012. “New Genetic Testing Reveals More Prenatal Abnormalities.” *Medical News Today*, December 7. Accessed February 20, 2013. www.medicalnewstoday.com/articles/253769.php.

Fixed: The Science/Fiction of Human Enhancement. 2013. Produced and Directed by Regan Brashear.

Fleck, Leonard M. 2009. *Just Caring: Health Care Rationing and Democratic Deliberation*. Oxford: Oxford University Press.

Fort Worth Star-Telegram. 2010. “Fort Worth Girl’s Starvation Death Prompts Arrests of her Mother, Sister.” *Dallas Morning News* September 22. Accessed June 15, 2014. http://www.dallasnews.com/news/community-news/fort-worth/headlines/20100922-Fort-Worth-girl-s-starvation-death-9852.ece

Foucault, Michel. 1973. *The Order of Things*. New York: Vintage Books.

———. 1977. "Nietzsche, Genealogy, History." In *Language, Counter-Memory, Practice: Selected Essays and Interviews by Michel Foucault*, edited by Donald F. Bouchard, translated by
Donald F. Bouchard and Sherry Simon, 139–164. Ithaca, NY: Cornell University Press.

———. 1979. *Discipline and Punish: The Birth of the Prison*. Translated by Alan Sheridan. New York: Random House.

———. 1980. "The Politics of Health in the Eighteenth Century." In *Power/Knowledge: Selected Interviews and Other Writings 1972–1977*, edited by Colin Gordon, translated by Colin Gordon, Leo Marshall, John Mepham, Kate Soper, 166–182. New York: Pantheon Books.

———. 1988. *Technologies of the Self: A Seminar with Michel Foucault*. Ed. Luther H. Martin, Huck Gutman, and Patrick H. Hutton. Amherst: The University of Massachusetts Press.

———. 1990. *The History of Sexuality, Volume 1: An Introduction*. Translated by Robert Hurley. New York: Vintage Books.

———. 2003a. *Abnormal: Lectures at the Collège de France, 1974–1975*. Edited by Valerio Marchetti and Antonella Salomoni. Translated by Graham Burchell. New York: Picador.

———.2003b. *"Society Must Be Defended": Lectures at the Collège de France, 1975–1976*. Edited by Mauro Bertani and Alessandro Fontana. Translated by David Macey. New York: Picador.

———. 2009. *Security, Territory, Population: Lectures at the Collège de France, 1977–1978*. Edited by Michel Senellart. Translated by Graham Burchell. New York: Picador.

———. 2010. *The Birth of Biopolitics: Lectures at the Collège de France, 1978–1979*. Edited by Michel Senellart. Translated by Graham Burchell. New York: Picador.

Francis, Leslie Pickering. 2009. "Understanding Autonomy in Light of Intellectual Disability." In *Disability and Disadvantage*, edited by Kimberley Brownlee and Adam Cureton, 200–215. Oxford: Oxford University Press.

Frank, Gelya. 2000. *Venus on Wheels: Two Decades of Dialogue on Disability, Biography, and Being Female in America*. Berkeley: University of California Press.

Franklin, Sarah. 1993. "Essentialism, Which Essentialism? Some Implications of Reproductive and Genetic Techno-Science." *Journal of Homosexuality* 24, No. 3–4: 27–40.

Fraser, Nancy and Linda Gordon. 2002. "A Genealogy of Dependency: Tracing a Keyword of the U.S. Welfare State." In *The Subject of Care: Feminist Perspectives on Dependency*, edited by Eva Feder Kittay and Ellen K. Feder, 14–39. New York: Rowman & Littlefield.

Fukuyama, Francis. 2002. *Our Posthuman Future: Consequences of the Biotechnology Revolution*. New York: Farrar, Straus, and Giroux.

———. 2004. "Transhumanism." *Foreign Policy* 144 (September–October): 42–43.

Gale, Sarah Fister. 2012. "Why Rick Santorum Would Have Killed My Daughter." *Jezebel* February 22. Accessed April 7, 2013. http://jezebel.com/5887417/why-rick-santorum-would-have-killed-my-daughter.

Garland-Thomson, Rosemarie. 1996. *Extraordinary Bodies: Figuring Disability in American Culture and Literature*. New York: Columbia University Press.

———. 2002. "Integrating Disability, Transforming Feminist Theory." *NWSA Journal* 14, No. 3: 1–32.

———. 2010. "Feminist Theory, the Body, and the Disabled Figure." In *The Disability Studies Reader*, edited by Lennard J. Davis, 279–294. New York: Routledge.

Garreau, Joel. 2005. *Radical Evolution: The Promise and Peril of Enhancing Our Minds, Our Bodies—and What It Means to Be Human*. New York: Doubleday.

Gattaca. 1997. DVD. Directed by Andrew Niccol. Culver City, CA: Columbia TriStar Home Video, 1998.

Gerber, Elaine. 2007. "Food Studies and Disability Studies: Introducing a Happy Marriage?" *Disability Studies Quarterly* 27, No. 3.

Glannon, Walter. 2008. "Decelerating and Arresting Human Aging." In *Medical Enhancement and Humanity*, edited by Bert Gordijn and Ruth Chadwick, 175–190. Springer.

Glenn, Cerise L. and Landra J. Cunningham. 2009. "The Power of Black Magic: The Magical Negro and White Salvation in Film." *Journal of Black Studies* 104, No. 4: 135–152.

Glover, Jonathan. 2006. *Choosing Children: Genes, Disability and Design*. New York: Oxford University Press.

———. 1984. *What Sort of People Should There Be? Genetic Engineering, Brain Control, and their Impact on Our Future World*. New York: Penguin Books.

Goering, Sara. 2008. "'You Say You're Happy, but…' Contested Quality of Life Judgments in Bioethics and Disability Studies." *Bioethical Inquiry* 5: 125–135.

Goffman, Erving. 1963. *Stigma: Notes on the Management of a Spoiled Identity*. New York: Simon & Schuster.

Gross, Zoe. 2012. "Killing Words." *Autistic Self Advocacy Network*, April 10. Accessed June 15, 2014. http://www.autisticadvocacy.org.

Gupta, Sanjay. 2012. "A Warning Against Genetic Testing." *CNN blogs*, April 2. Accessed May 1, 2012. http://thechart.blogs.cnn.com/2012/04/02/a-warning-against-genetic testing/?hpt=hp_bn12.

Habermas, Jürgen. 2003. *The Future of Human Nature: On the Way to a Liberal Eugenics?* Translated by Hella Beister and William Rehg. Cambridge, UK: Polity Press.

Hall, Melinda. 2013. "Vile Sovereigns in Bioethical Debate." *Disability Studies Quarterly* 33, No. 4. Accessed July 31, 2016. doi: 0.18061/dsq.v33i4.3870.

———. 2016. "Horrible Heroes: Liberating Alternative Visions of Disability in Horror." *Disability Studies Quarterly* 36, No. 1. Accessed July 31, 2016. doi: 10.18061/dsq.v36i1.3258.

Haraway, Donna. 1991. *Simians, Cyborgs, and Women: The Reinvention of Nature*. New York: Routledge.

Harris, John. 1992. *Wonderwoman and Superman: The Ethics of Human Biotechnology*. New York: Oxford University Press.

———. 2004. "Immortal Ethics." In *Annals N Y Acad Sci.* 1019: 527–534.

———. 2007. *Enhancing Evolution: The Ethical Case for Making Better People*. Princeton, NJ: Princeton University Press.

———. 2011. "Enhancements are a Moral Obligation." In *Human Enhancement*, edited by Julian Savulescu and Nick Bostrom. Oxford, UK: Oxford University Press.

Hartley, Christie. 2009a. "An Inclusive Contractualism: Obligations to the Mentally Disabled." In *Disability and Disadvantage*, edited by Kimberley Brownlee and Adam Cureton: 138–162. Oxford: Oxford University Press.

———. 2009b. "Justice for the Disabled: A Contractualist Approach." *Journal of Social Philosophy* 40, No. 1: 17–36.

———. 2011. "Disability and Justice." *Philosophy Compass* 6, No. 2: 120–132.

Haslam, Nick. 2011. "Genetic Essentialism, Neuroessentialism, and Stigma: Commentary on Dar-Nimrod and Heine." *Psychological Bulletin* 137, No. 5: 819–824.

Hauskeller, Michael. 2012. "Reinventing Cockaigne: Utopian Themes in Transhumanist Thought." *Hastings Center Report* 42, No. 2: 39–47.

Hayles, N. Katherine. 1999. *How We Became Posthuman: Virtual Bodies in Cybernetics, Literature, and Informatics.* Chicago: University of Chicago Press.

Heard, Alex. 1997. "Technology Makes Us Optimistic; They Want To Live." *The New York Times Magazine*, September 28. Accessed January 28, 2012. Academic OneFile. Web.

Heasley, Shaun. 2012. "Parents Sue for Millions after Daughter Born with Down syndrome." *The Disability Scoop*, March 2. Accessed March 2. http://www.disabilityscoop.com/2012/03/02/parents-sue-downsyndrome/15100/.

———. 2013. "Autism Rate Soars to 1 in 50 Kids." *Disability Scoop* March 20. Accessed March 26. http://www.disabilityscoop.com/2013/03/20/autism-rate-1-in-50/17540/.

———. 2013. "Soon To Be Wed, Couple With Disabilities Sue to Live Together." *Disability Scoop* April 2. Accessed April 10. http://www.disabilityscoop.com/2013/04/04/soon-wed-sue-live/17646/.

Hershey, Laura. 1994. *Ms. Magazine* (July/August).

Hill, Erica. 2012. "Early Prenatal Test Raises Ethical Questions." *CBS News* Feb 22. Accessed March 1, 2012: www.cbsnews.com/8301–505269_162–57382535/early-prenatal-test-raises-ethical-questions/.

Hof, Robert. 2014. "Seven Months After FDA Slapdown, 23andMe Returns with New Health Report Submission." *Forbes*, June 20. Accessed November 2, 2015. http://www.forbes.com/sites/roberthof/2014/06/20/seven-months-after-fda-slapdown-23andme-returns-with-new-health-report-submission/.

Hoffman, Diane E. and Anita J. Tarzian. 2001. "The Girl Who Cried Pain: A Bias Against Women in the Treatment of Pain." *Journal of Law, Medicine & Ethics* 29: 13–27.

Holden, Constance. 1997. "Didactics of Gattaca." *Science* November 7: 1019.

hooks, bell. 1995. *Killing Rage: Ending Racism.* New York: Henry Holt and Company.

Hubbard, Ruth. 2010. "Abortion and Disability: Who Should and Should Not Inhabit the World?" In *The Disability Studies Reader*, edited by Lennard J. Davis, 107–119. New York: Routledge.

Hughes, James. 1996. "Embracing Change with All Four Arms: A Post-Humanist Defense of Genetic Engineering." *Eubios: Journal of Asian and International Bioethics* 6, No. 4: 94–101.

———. 2001. "The Future of Death: Cryonics and the Telos of Liberal Individualism." *Journal of Evolution and Technology* 6 (July).

———. 2004. *Citizen Cyborg: Why Democratic Societies Must Respond to the Redesigned Human of the Future*. New York: Basic Books.

———. 2007a. "Becoming a Better Person." *TransVision Lecture*. Accessed July 13, 2013 .http://www.transhumanismi.org/tv06/presentations/James%20Hughes%20-%20Moral%20Cognition.pdf.

———. 2007b. "Human vs. Posthuman." *Hastings Center Report* 37, No. 5: 4–7.

———. 2007c. "The Struggle for a Smarter World." *Futures* 39: 942–954.

———. 2009. "Battle Plan to Be More Than Well: Transhumanism is finally getting in gear." August 6. Accessed June 29, 2016. http://www.transhumanism.org/index.php/th/more/509/.*humanity* +. 2012. "Transhumanist FAQ." Accessed August 31. http://humanityplus.org/philosophy/transhumanist-faq/.

Hurley, Dan. 1985. "Arresting Delinquency." *Psychology Today (*March): 63.

Huxley, Aldous. 1931. *Brave New World*. London: Chatto & Windus.

———. 1939. *After Many a Summer Dies the Swan*. Harper & Row.

Huxley, Julian. 1948. *Man in the Modern World*. New York: New American Library.

———. 1927. *Religion Without Revelation*. London: Ernest Benn.

Ida, Ryuichi. 2011. "Should We Improve Human Nature? An Interrogation from an Asian Perspective." In *Human Enhancement*, edited by Julian Savulescu and Nick Bostrom, 59–70. Oxford, UK: Oxford University Press.

Ingus-Arkell, Esther. 2012. "How to Build the Perfect Human." *i09* Feb 15. Accessed March 23. http://io9.com/5885222/what-would-be-the-perfect-combination-of-animal-powers-to-have.

InteliHealth. 2014. "Fragile X Genetic Testing Basics." In cooperation with Harvard Medical School. Accessed June 20.www.intelihealth.com.

Iwakuma, Miho. 2002. "The Body as Embodiment: An Investigation of the Body by Merleau-Ponty." In *Disability/Postmodernity: Embodying Disability Theory*, edited by Mairian Corker and Tom Shakespeare, 76–87. London: Continuum Press.

James, Susan Donaldson. 2009. "Down Syndrome Births are Down in the U.S." *ABC News* Nov 2. Accessed September 1, 2012. http://abcnews.go.com/Health/w_ParentingResource/down-syndrome-births-drop-us-women-abort/story?id=8960803#.UDA-9N2PWqM.

"Jerry Lewis Responds to Critics at Opening of 26th Telethon." 1991. *Los Angeles Times* September 2. Accessed October 7. articles.latimes.com/1991–09–02/news/mn-1155_1_jerry-lewis.

Johnson, Harriet McBryde. 2003. "Should I have Been Killed at Birth? The Case for My Life." *New York Times Magazine* February 16.

Juengst, Eric. 1998. "What Does Enhancement Mean?" In *Enhancing Human Traits: Ethical and Social Implications*, edited by Erik Parens, 29–47. Washington, DC: Georgetown University Press.

Kafer, Alison. 2011. "Debating Feminist Futures: Slippery Slopes, Cultural Anxiety, and the Case of the Deaf Lesbians." In *Feminist Disability Studies,* edited by Kim Q. Hall, 218–242. Indianapolis: Indiana University Press.

Kass, Leon. 1997. "The Wisdom of Repugnance." *The New Republic* 216, No. 22: 17–26.

———. 1999. "The Moral Meaning of Genetic Technology." *Commentary* 108, No. 2: 32–38.

———. 2002. *Life, Liberty and the Pursuit of Dignity*. San Francisco: Encounter Books.

———. 2007. "Deeper Disquiets with Biotechnological Enhancement." Presented at Harvard Law School, March 17.

Keller, Evelyn Fox. 1992. *Secrets of Life, Secrets of Death: Essays on Language, Gender and Science*. New York: Routledge.

———. 2000. *The Century of the Gene*. Cambridge, MA: Harvard University Press.

Keller, Evelyn Fox and Helen E. Longino. 1996. *Feminism and Science*. Oxford: Oxford University Press.

Keller, Johannes. 2005. "In Genes We Trust: The Biological Component of Psychological Essentialism and Its Relationship to Mechanisms of Motivated Social Cognition." *Journal of Personality and Social Psychology* 88, No. 4: 686–702.

Kelly, Christine. 2010. "Wrestling with Group Identity: Disability Activism and Direct Funding." *Disability Studies Quarterly* 30, No. 3/4.

Kennedy, Kelli. 2012. "Feds: Thousands of Disabled Florida kids May End Up in Nursing Homes." *Orlando Sentinel*, September 8. Accessed October 5.http://articles.orlandosentinel.com/2012–0908/health/os-disabled-kids-nursing-homes-florida-lawsuit-20120907 _1_americans-with-disabilities-act-florida-pam-bondi?pagewanted=all.

Kerr, Anne and Tom Shakespeare. 2002. *Genetic Politics: From Eugenics to Genome*. Gretton, UK: New Clarion Press.

Kevles, Daniel. 1985. *In the Name of Eugenics*. Berkeley and Los Angeles: University of California Press.

———. 2003. "Science and the Deconstruction of Human Nature." In *The Future of Human Nature: a Symposium on the Promises and Challenges of the Revolutions in Genomics and Computer Science*, edited by Charles DeLisi and Kenneth Lewes, 33–36. Boston University: Frederick S. Pardee Center for the Study of the Longer-Range Future.

Kevles, Daniel and Leroy Hood, eds. 1993. *The Code of Codes: Scientific and Social Issues in the Human Genome Project*. Cambridge: Harvard University Press.

Khavari, David A., George L. Sen, and John L. Rinn. "DNA Methylation and Epigenetic Control of Cellular Differentiation." Cell Cycle 9.19 (2010): 3880–3883.

"KidsHealth: Genetic Counseling." 2012. *Nemours*. Accessed July 23. http://kidshealth.org/parent/system/medical/genetic_counseling.html.

Kittay, Eva Feder. 1999. *Love's Labor: Essays on Women, Equality and Dependency*. New York: Routledge.

———. 2000a. "On the Expressivity and Ethics of Selective Abortion for Disability: Conversations with My Son." In *Prenatal Testing and Disability Rights*, edited by Erik Parens and Adrienne Asch, 165–198. Washington, DC: Georgetown University Press.

———. 2000b. "Rationality, Personhood, and Peter Singer on the Fate of Severely Impaired Infants." *APA Newsletter on Philosophy and Medicine* 99, No. 2 (Spring).

———. 2001. "When Caring is Just and Justice is Caring: Justice and Mental Retardation." *Public Culture* 13, No. 3: 557–579.

———. 2006. "Thoughts on the Desire for Normality." In *Surgically Shaping Children: Technology, Ethics, and the Pursuit of Normality*, edited by Erik Parens, 90–110. Baltimore: Johns Hopkins University Press.

———. 2009. "The Ethics of Philosophizing." In *Feminist Ethics and Social and Political Philosophy: Theorizing the Non-Ideal*, edited by Lisa Tessman: 121–146. Springer.

———. 2010a. "Lives Not Worth Living: Mental Disability, Race, and the Nazi's T-4 Project." Philosophy in an Inclusive Key Summer Institute, Pennsylvania State University July 29. Presentation.

———. 2010b. "The Personal is Philosophical Is Political: A Philosopher and Mother of a Cognitively Disabled Person Sends Notes from the Battlefield." In *Cognitive Disability and Its Challenge to Moral Philosophy*, edited by Eva Feder Kittay and Licia Carlson, 393–413. Wiley-Blackwell.

———. 2010c. "Planning a Trip to Italy, Arriving in Holland: The Delusion of Choice in Planning a Family." *International Journal of Feminist Approaches to Bioethics* 3, No. 2: 9–24.

Kittay, Eva and Ellen Feder. 2002. *The Subject of Care: Feminist Perspectives on Dependency*. New York: Rowman & Littlefield.

Klitzman, Robert. 2012. *Am I My Genes? Confronting Fate and Family Secrets in the Age of Genetic Testing*. Oxford: Oxford University Press.

Koch, Tom. 2004. "The Difference that Difference Makes: Bioethics and the Challenge of 'disability,'" *Journal of Medicine and Philosophy* 29: 697–716.

———. 2006. "Bioethics as Ideology: Conditional and Unconditional Values." *Journal of Medicine and Philosophy* 31: 251–267.

———. 2010. "Enhancing Who? Enhancing What? Ethics, Bioethics, and Transhumanism." *Journal of Medicine and Philosophy* 35: 685–699.

Kolata, Gina. 2012. "Study says DNA's Power to Predict Illness is Limited." *The New York Times* April 2. Accessed May 1, 2012. http://www.nytimes.com/2012/04/03/health/research/dnas-power-to-predict-is-limited-study-finds.html.

Kramer, Peter D. 1993. *Listening to Prozac*. New York: Viking Press.

Kristiansen, Kristjana, Simo Vehmas, and Tom Shakespeare, eds. 2009. *Arguing about Disability: Philosophical Perspectives*. New York: Routledge.

Kröner, Hans-Peter. 1999. "From Eugenics to Genetic Screening: Historical Problems of Human Genetic Applications." In *The Ethics of Genetic Screening,* edited by Ruth Chadwick, Darren Schickle, Henk ten Have, and Urban Wiesing, 131–145. The Netherlands: Kluwer Academic Publishers.

Kuppers, Petra. 2006. "Disability Culture Poetry: The Sound of the Bones. A Literary Essay." *Disability Studies Quarterly* 26, No. 4.

Kurzweil, Ray. 2000. *The Age of Spiritual Machines: When Computers Exceed Human Intelligence*. New York: Penguin Books.

———. 2006. *The Singularity is Near: When Humans Transcend Biology*. New York: Viking Press, Penguin Books.

Kurzweil, Ray and Terry Grossman. 2010. *Transcend: Nine Steps to Living Well Forever*. Rodale.

Lagu, Tara et al. 2013. "Access to Subspecialty Care for Patients with Mobility Impairment: A Survey." *Annals of Internal Medicine* 158: 441–446.

Lane, Harlan. 2010. "Construction of Deafness." In *The Disability Studies Reader*, edited by Lennard J. Davis, 77–93. New York: Routledge.

Lauritzen, Paul. 1995. "Whose Bodies? Which Selves? Appeals to Embodiment in Assessments of Reproductive Technology." In *Embodiment, Morality, and Medicine*, edited by L. Sowle Cahill and M.A. Farley, 113–126. Dordrecht, The Netherlands: Kluwer.

Lemke, Thomas. 2011. *Bio-Politics: An Advanced Introduction*. New York: New York University Press.

Lewontin, Richard C. 1992. *Biology as Ideology*. New York: Harper.

Liao, S. Matthew, Anders Sandberg, and Rebecca Roache. 2012. "Human Engineering and Climate Change." *Ethics, Policy, and the Environment* 15 (2): 206–221.

Liggett, Helen. 1988. "Stars are not Born: An Interpretive Approach to the Politics of Disability." *Disability, Handicap and Society* 3, No. 3: 263–276.

Lippman, Abby. 1991. "Prenatal Testing and Screening: Constructing Needs and Reinforcing Inequities." *American Journal of Law and Medicine* 17, No. 1–2: 15–50.

———. 1993. "Prenatal Genetic Testing and Geneticization: Mother Matters for All." *Fetal DiagnTher* 8, supplement 1: 175–88.

Little, Margaret Olivia. 1998. "Cosmetic Surgery, Suspect Norms, and the Ethics of Complicity." In *Enhancing Human Traits: Ethical and Social Implications*, edited by Erik Parens, 162-176. Washington, DC: Georgetown University Press.

Littlefield, Dana. 2012. "Mother Admitted Killing Son to Police." *The San Diego Union Tribune* April 4. Accessed June 18, 2014. http://www.utsandiego.com.

Lobo, Ingrid. 2008. "Birth Defects: Prevention and Treatment." *Nature Education* 1, No. 1: n. pag. Web.

Longmore, Paul K. 1987. "Screening Stereotypes: Images of Disabled People in Television and Motion Pictures." In *Images of the Disabled, Disabling Images*, edited by Allan Gartner and Tom Joe. New York: Praeger.

Lotz, Mianna. 2008. "Overstating the Biological: Geneticism and Essentialism in Social Cloning and Social Sex Selection." In *The Sorting Society: The Ethics of Genetic Screening and Therapy*, edited by Janna Thompson and Loane Skene, 133–148. Cambridge: Cambridge University Press.

Loughlin, Michael. 1995. "Bioethics and the Mythology of Liberalism." *Health Care Analysis* 3: 315–323.

Machiavelli, Niccolò. 1950. *The Prince and the Discourses*. New York: Random House.

Mackenzie, Catriona and Jackie Leach Scully. 2007. "Moral Imagination, Disability and Embodiment." *Journal of Applied Philosophy* 24, No. 4: 335–351.

Mansfield, Caroline, Suellen Hopfer and Theresa M. Marteau. 1999. "Termination Rates After Prenatal Diagnosis of Down syndrome, Spina Bifida, Anencephaly, and Turner and Klinefelter Syndromes: A Systematic Literature Review." *Prenatal Diagnosis* 19: 808–812.

Meyer-Rochow, V. B. 2009. "Food taboos: Their origins and purposes." *Journal of Ethnobiologyand Ethnomedicine* 5: 18–27.

Meyers, Diana Tietjens. 2005. "Decentralizing Autonomy: Five Faces of Selfhood." In *Autonomy and the Challenges to Liberalism: New Essays*, edited by John Christman and Joel Anderson, 27–55. Cambridge, UK: Cambridge University Press.

McMahan, Jeff. 2003. *The Ethics of Killing*. Oxford: Oxford University Press.

———. 2005. "Preventing the Existence of People with Disabilities." In *Quality of Life and Human Difference: Genetic Testing, Health Care, and Disability*, edited by David Wasserman, Jerome Bickenbach, and Robert Wachbroit, 142–171. Cambridge: Cambridge University Press.

———. 2010. "Cognitive Disability and Cognitive Enhancement." In *Cognitive Disability and Its Challenge to Moral Philosophy*, edited by Eva Feder Kittay and Licia Carlson, 345–368. Wiley-Blackwell.

McNally, Ruth and Peter Glasner. 2006. "Survival of the Gene? 21st-Century Visions from Genomics, Proteomics and the New Biology." In *New Genetics, New Social Formations*, edited by Peter Glasner, Paul Atkinson, and Helen Greenslade, 253–278. Taylor & Francis.

McRuer, Robert. 2006. *Crip Theory: Cultural Signs of Queerness and Disability*. New York: New York University Press.

Mehlman, Maxwell and Jeffrey Botkin. 1998. *Access to the Genome: The Challenge to Equality*.Washington, DC: Georgetown University Press.

Mendieta, Eduardo. 2003. "We Have Never Been Human, or, How We Lost Our Humanity: Derrida and Habermas on Cloning." *Philosophy Today* 47: 168–175.

Miko, Ilona. 2008. "Phenotype Variability: Penetrance and Expressivity." *Nature Education* 1, No. 1.

Miles, Kathleen. 2013. "'Fat Genes' Determine Obesity, UCLA Study Says, In Addition To Diet And Exercise." *The Huffington Post*, January 10. Accessed March 26. http://www.huffingtonpost.com/2013/01/10/fat-genes-obesity-ucla-study-diet-exercise_n_2450108.html.

Mills, Catherine. 2011. *Futures of Reproduction: Bioethics and Biopolitics*. Springer.

Mills, Claudia. 2003. "The Child's Right to an Open Future?" *Journal of Social Philosophy* 34, No. 4 (Winter): 499–509.

Mintz, Susannah B. 2007. *Unruly Bodies: Life Writing by Women with Disabilities*. Chapel Hill: The University of North Carolina Press.

Mitchell, David T. and Sharon L. 2000. *Narrative Prosthesis: Disability and the Dependencies of Discourse*. Ann Arbor: University of Michigan Press.

Mitra, Monika, Karen Clements, Jianying Zhang, Lisa Iezzoni, Suzanne Smeltzer, and Linda Long-Bellil. 2015. "Maternal Characteristics, Pregnancy Complications, and Adverse Birth Outcomes Among Women with Disabilities." *Medical Care* 53, No. 12: 1027–1032.

Montgomery, Cal. 1999. "A Defense of Genocide." *Ragged Edge Online* July/August. Last Accessed September 4, 2012:http://www.raggededgemagazine.com/0799/b799ps.htm.

Morris, Jenny. 1991. *Pride Against Prejudice*. London: Women's Press.

Morrison, Daniel R. 2008. "Making the Autonomous Client: How Genetic Counselors Construct Autonomous Subjects." In *Bioethical Issues, Sociological Perspectives*, edited by Barbara Katz Rothman, Elizabeth Mitchell Armstrong, and Rebecca Tiger, 179–198. Amsterdam/London: Elsevier.

Moyer, Jeff (Producer), and Judy Leasure (Executive Producer). 2004. CD. *Lest We Forget*. Highland Heights, OH & Dayton, OH: Music from the Heart and Partners for Community Living.

Moyer, Jeff. 2007. "Food and Hunger. Transcript from CD, entitled "*LEST WE FORGET…,*"Track 33: Food and Hunger." *Disability Studies Quarterly* 27 No. 3: n. pag.

———. 2013. "Music from the Heart: Jeff Moyer." *Jeffmoyer.com*. Web.

Mullins, Aimee. 2009. "My 12 pairs of legs." *TED*. Accessed July 30, 2016. https://www.ted.com/talks/aimee_mullins_prosthetic_aesthetics?language=en.

Munch, Shari. 2004. "Gender-Biased Diagnosing of Women's Medical Complaints: Contributions of Feminist Thought, 1970–1995." *Women & Health* 40, No.1: 101–121.

Murphy, Amy O., Robbie M. Sutton, Karen M. Douglas and Leigh M. McLellan. 2011. "Ambivalent Sexism and the 'do's' and 'don'ts" of Pregnancy: Examining Attitudes Toward Proscriptions and the Women Who Flout Them." *Personality and Individual Differences* 51: 812–816.

"National Society to Conserve Life: Life Extension Institute Formed to Teach Hygiene and Prevention of Disease." *The New York Times* December 30, 1913.

Nelkin, Dorothy and M. Susan Lindee. 1995. *The DNA Mystique: The Gene as a Cultural Icon*. New York: W. H. Freeman and Company.

Nelson, James Lindemann. 2000. "The Meaning of the Act: Reflections on the Expressive Force of Reproductive Decision Making and Policies." In *Prenatal Testing and Disability Rights*, edited by Erik Parens and Adrienne Asch, 196–213. Washington, DC: Georgetown University Press.

———. 2007. "Synecdoche and Stigma." *Cambridge Quarterly of Healthcare Ethics* 16: 478.

———. 2011. "Hurts, Insults, and Stigmas: A Comment on Murphy." *Journal of Medical Ethics* 37, No. 2: 66–67.

Nozick, Robert. 1974. *Anarchy, State and Utopia*. New York: Basic Books.

Nussbaum, Martha. 2002. "The Future of Feminist Liberalism." In *The Subject of Care: Feminist Perspectives on Dependency*, edited by Eva Feder Kittay and Ellen K. Feder, 186–214. New York: Rowman & Littlefield.

———. 2007. *Frontiers of Justice: Disability, Nationality, Species Membership*. Cambridge: Harvard University Press.

O'Brien, Ruth. 2005. *Bodies in Revolt: Gender, Disability, and a Workplace Ethic of Care*. New York: Routledge.

O'Mathúna, Dónal P. 2009. *Nanoethics: Big Ethical Issues with Small Technology*. New York: Continuum.

Oliver, Kelly. 2002. "Subjectivity as Responsivity: The Ethical Implications of Dependency." In *The Subject of Care: Feminist Perspectives on Dependency*, edited by Eva Kittay and Ellen Feder, 322–333. New York: Rowman & Littlefield.

———. 2010. "Enhancing Evolution: Whose Body? Whose Choice?" *Southern Journal of Philosophy* 48, Spindel supplement (September): 74–96.

———. 2011. "Deconstructing 'Grown versus Made': A Derridean Perspective on Cloning." *Journal of Philosophy: A Cross-Disciplinary Inquiry* 7, No. 16 (Fall): 45–52.

———. 2013. *Technologies of Life and Death: From Cloning to Capital Punishment.* Fordham University Press.

Overall, Christine. 1987. *Ethics and Human Reproduction: A Feminist Analysis.* Boston: Allen & Unwin.

———. 1993. *Human Reproduction: Principles, Practices, Policies.* Oxford: Oxford University Press.

———. 2012. *Why Have Children?* Cambridge: MIT Press.

Parens, Erik. 1995. "The Goodness of Fragility: On the Prospect of Genetic Technologies Aimed at the Enhancement of Human Capacities." *Kennedy Institute of Ethics Journal* 5, No. 2: 141–153.

———. ed. 1998. *Enhancing Human Traits: Ethical and Social Implications.* Washington, DC: Georgetown University Press.

———. ed. 2006. *Surgically Shaping Children: Technology, Ethics, and the Pursuit of Normality.* Baltimore: Johns Hopkins University Press.

———. 2008. "Puzzling about Peter Singer." *The Hastings Center Report* 38, No. 6 (Field Notes).

———. 2009. "Toward a More Fruitful Debate About Enhancement." In *Human Enhancement*, edited by Julian Savulescu and Nick Bostrom, 181–197. Oxford, UK: Oxford University Press.

Parens, Erik and Adrienne Asch, eds. 2000. *Prenatal Testing and Disability Rights.* Washington, DC: Georgetown University Press.

Parfit, Derek. 1984. *Reasons and Persons.* Oxford, UK: Oxford University Press.

Passmore, John. 1970. *The Perfectibility of Man.* New York: Charles Scribner's Sons.

Pauer-Studer, Herlinde. 2006. "Public Reason and Bioethics." *Medscape General Medicine* 8, No. 4: 13.

Paul, Diane. 1995. *Controlling Human Heredity, 1865 to the Present.* Atlantic Highlands, NJ: Humanities Press.

Puar, Jasbir. 2009. "Prognosis time: Towards a geopolitics of affect, debility and capacity." *Women & Peformance: a journal of feminist theory* 19, No. 2: 161–172.

Peace, William. 2012. "Comfort Care as Denial of Personhood." *Hastings Center Report* 42, No. 4: 14–17.

———. 2013a. "Euthanasia in Belgium: The Untold Story." *Bioethics Forum* February 2. Last Accessed April 9, 2013: http://www.thehastingscenter.org/Bioethicsforum/Post.aspx?id=6222&blogid=140.

———. 2013b. "A Peaceful Death or a Risk to People with Disabilities?" *Bioethics Forum* March 19. Accessed April 9. http://www.thehastingscenter.org/Bioethicsforum/Post.aspx?id=6285&blogid=140.

Pearson, Helen. 2009. "One Gene, Twenty Years." *Nature* 460 (July 8): 164–149.

Perine, Shawn. 2011. "Your Physique: National Health and Physical Culture Magazine." *Flex* 29, No. 1: 60.

Persson, Ingmar and Julian Savulescu. 2010. "Moral Transhumanism." *Journal of Medicine and Philosophy* 35: 656–669.

———. 2012. *Unfit for the Future: The Need for Moral Enhancement.* Oxford: Oxford University Press.

Physical Culture (Magazine). 1899–1950. Bernarr Macfadden.

Piepmeier, Alison. 2012. "Choosing to Have a Child with Down Syndrome." *The New York Times*, March 2. Accessed March 26, 2013. http://parenting.blogs.nytimes.com/2012/03/02/choosing-to-have-a-child-with-down-syndrome/.

Pinker, Steven. 2004. "Can We Change Human Nature?" In *The Future of Human Nature: A Symposium on the Promises and Challenges of the Revolutions in Genomics and Computer Science*, edited by Charles DeLisi and Kenneth Lewes, 25–28. Boston University: Frederick S. Pardee Center for the Study of the Longer-Range Future.

Piore, Adam. 2014. "The Neuroscientist Who Wants to Upload Humanity to a Computer." *Popular Science* April 10. Accessed April 17. http://www.popsci.com/article/science/neuroscientist-who-wants-upload-humanity-computer.

Proctor, Robert. 1988. *Racial Hygiene: Medicine Under the Nazis*. Cambridge, MA: Harvard University Press.

Radick, Gregory. 2001. "The Century of the Gene." *Heredity* 86: 639–64. *A Ragged Edge Online*. Accessed April 6, 2013. www.ragged-edge-mag.com.

Ralston, Steven J. 2000. "Reflections from the Trenches: One Doctor's Encounter with Disability Rights Arguments." In *Prenatal Testing and Disability Rights*, edited by Erik Parens and Adrienne Asch, 334–390. Washington, DC: Georgetown University Press.

Ramsey, Paul. 1970. *Fabricated Man*. Yale.

Rapp, Rayna. 1998. "Chromosomes and Communication: The Discourse of Genetic Counseling." *Medical Anthropology Quarterly* 2: 143–157.

Rawls, John. 2007. *Lectures on the History of Political Philosophy*. Edited by Samuel Freeman. Cambridge: Belknap Press.

———. 1996. *Political Liberalism*. New York: Columbia University Press.

———. 1997. "The Idea of Public Reason Revisited." *The University of Chicago Law Review* 64, No. 3 (Summer): 765–807.

———. 1999. *A Theory of Justice: Revised Edition*. Cambridge: Belknap Press.

Reik, Wolf. 2007. "Stability and Flexibility of Epigenetic Gene Regulation in Mammalian Development." *Nature* 447, No. 7143: 425–32.

Reinders, Hans S. 2000. *The Future of the Disabled in Liberal Society: An Ethical Analysis*. Notre Dame, IN: University of Notre Dame Press.

Resnik, David B. and Daniel B. Vorhaus. 2006. "Genetic Modification and Genetic Determinism." *Philosophy, Ethics, and Humanities in Medicine* 1: 9.

Riis, Jason, George Loewenstein, Jonathan Baron, Christopher Jepson, Angela Fagerlin, and Peter A. Ubel. 2005. "Ignorance of Hedonic Adaptation to Hemodialysis: A Study Using Ecological Momentary Assessment." *Journal of Experimental Psychology* 134, No. 1: 3-9.

Riley, Charles A. 2005. *Disability and the Media: Prescriptions for Change*. Hanover: University Press of New England.

Riley, Denise. 1998. *Am I That Name?* Basingstoke: Macmillan.

Robison, John Elder. 2008. *Look Me in the Eye: My Life with Asperger's*. Three Rivers Press.

Rogers, Lois. 1999. "Having Disabled Babies Will be 'sin' Says Scientist." *Sunday Times* (London) July 4. Accessed April 6, 2013. https://www.jiscmail.ac.uk/cgi-bin/webadmin?A2=disability-research;4c00879.9907.

Rohrer, Judy. 2005. "Toward a Full-Inclusion Feminism: A Feminist Deployment of Disability Analysis." *Feminist Studies* 31, No. 1: 34–63.

Rose, Hilary. 1994. "Feminism and the Genetic Turn: Challenging Reproductive Technoscience." In *Love, Power and Knowledge: Towards a Feminist Transformation of the Sciences*, 172–207. Bloomington: Indiana University Press.

Rothman, Sheila M. and David J. Rothman J. 2003. *The Pursuit of Perfection: The Promise and Perils of Medical Enhancement.* New York: Pantheon Books.

Rubin, Charles T. 2008. "What is the Good of Transhumanism?" In *Medical Enhancement and Humanity*, edited by Bert Gordijn and Ruth Chadwick: 137–156. Springer.

Salem, Tania. 1999. "Physician-Assisted Suicide: Promoting Autonomy—or Medicalizing Suicide?" *The Hastings Center Report* 29 (3): 30–36.

Sandberg, Anders and Nick Bostrom. 2006. "Converging Cognitive Enhancements." *Ann. N.Y. Acad. Sci.* 1093: 201–227.

Sandel, Michael J. 2004. "The Case Against Perfection." *The Atlantic Monthly* 293, No. 3: 51–62.

———. 2007. *The Case Against Perfection: Ethics in the Age of Genetic Engineering*. Cambridge, MA: Harvard University Press.

Sanford, Emily Sullivan. 2006. "My Shoe Size Stayed the Same: Maintaining a Positive Sense of Identity with Achondroplasia and Limb-Lengthening Surgeries." In *Surgically Shaping Children: Technology, Ethics, and the Pursuit of Normality*, edited by Erik Parens, 29–42. Baltimore: Johns Hopkins University Press.

Savulescu, Julian. 2001a. "In Defense of Selection for Non-Disease Genes." *The American Journal of Bioethics* 1, No. 1 (Winter): 16–19.

———. 2001b. "Procreative Beneficence: Why We Should Select the Best Children." *Bioethics* 15, No. 5–6: 413–426.

———. 2001c. "Resources, Down's Syndrome, and Cardiac Surgery: Do We Really Want Equality of Access?" *BMJ* 322, No. 7291 (April 14): 875–876.

———. 2002. "Deaf Lesbians, 'Designer Disability,' and the Future of Medicine." *BMJ* 325, No. 7367 (October 5): 771–773.

———. 2009. "Genetically Enhance Humanity or Face Extinction." *Festival of Dangerous Ideas, Sydney Opera House*, October. Accessed August 31, 2012. http://www.themonthly.com.au/genetically-enhance-humanity-or-face-extinction-julian-savulescu-2065.

Savulescu, Julian and Nick Bostrom, eds. 2011. *Human Enhancement.* Oxford, UK: Oxford University Press.

Savulescu, Julian and Guy Kahane. 2009. "The Moral Obligation to Create Children with the Best Chance of the Best Life." *Bioethics* 23, No. 5: 274–290.

Savulescu, Julian, Melanie Hemsley, Ainsley Newson, and Bennett Foddy. 2006. "Behavioural Genetics: Why Eugenic Selection is Preferable to Enhancement." *Journal of Applied Philosophy* 23, No. 2: 157–171.

Savulescu, Julian, Ruud ter Meulen, and Guy Kahane, eds. 2010. *Enhancing Human Capacities*. Oxford: Wiley-Blackwell.

Sawicki, Jana. 1994. "Foucault, Feminism and Questions of Identity." In *The Cambridge Companion to Foucault*, edited by Gary Gutting: 286–313. Cambridge: Cambridge University Press.

Saxton, Marsha. 2000. "Why Members of the Disability Community Oppose Prenatal Diagnosis and Selective Abortion." In *Prenatal Testing and Disability Rights*, edited by Erik Parens and Adrienne Asch, 147–164. Washington, DC: Georgetown University Press.

Scheer, Jessica and Nora Groce. 1998. "Impairment as a Human Constant: Cross-Cultural and Historical Perspectives on Variation," *Journal of Social Issues* 44: 23–37.

Schweik, Susan. 2010. *The Ugly Laws: Disability in Public*. New York: NYU Press.

Scott-Hill, Mairian, 2004. "Collectivising Experience and Rules of Engagement: Close(d) Encounters in Disability Research." In *Implementing the Social Model of Disability: Theory and Research*, edited by C. Barnes and G. Mercer, 157–171. Leeds: The Disability Press.

Scully, Jackie Leach. 2001. "Drawing a Line: Situating Moral Boundaries in Genetic Medicine." *Bioethics* 15, No. 3: 189–204.

———. 2002. "A Postmodern Disorder: Moral Encounters with Molecular Models of Disability." In *Disability/Postmodernity: Embodying Political Theory*, edited by Marian Corker and Tom Shakespeare, 48–61. London: Continuum.

———. 2008. *Disability Bioethics: Moral Bodies, Moral Difference*. Lanham, MD: Rowman & Littlefield Publishers, Inc.

———. 2012. "Disability, Human Rights and Contemporary Genetics." *eLS*. Chichester: John Wiley & Sons, Ltd. doi: 10.1002/9780470015902.a0005214.pub2.

Shakespeare, Tom. 2006. *Disability Rights and Wrongs*. Taylor & Francis.

Shakespeare, Tom and Mark Erickson. 2001. "Different Strokes: Beyond Biological Determinism and Social Constructionism." In *Alas Poor Darwin: Arguments Against Evolutionary Psychology*, edited by Hilary Rose and Steven Rose, 190–205. New York: Vintage.

Shapiro, Joseph P. 1994. *No Pity: People with Disabilities Forging a New Civil Rights Movement*. New York: Random House.

Shapshay, Sandra. 2009. "Lifting the Genetic Veil of Ignorance: Is There Anything Really Unjust about Gattacan Society?" In *Bioethics at the Movies*, edited by Sandra Shapshay, 87–101. Baltimore: The Johns Hopkins University Press.

Shiffrin, Seana Valentine. 1999. "Wrongful Life, Procreative Responsibility, and the Significance of Harm." *Legal Theory* 5: 117–148.

Shostak, Stanley. 2002. *Becoming Immortal: Combining Cloning and Stem-Cell Therapy*. New York: SUNY Press.

Siever, Larry. 1997. *The New View of the Self: How Genes and Neurotransmitters Shape Your Mind, Personality and Your Mental Health*. Old Tappan, NJ: Macmillan.

Silver, Lee. 2004. "The Inevitability of Human Genetic Enhancement and its Impact on Humanity." In *The Future of Human Nature: a Symposium on the Promises and Challenges of the Revolutions in Genomics and Computer Science*, edited by Charles DeLisi and Kenneth Lewes, 12–15. Boston University: Frederick S. Pardee Center for the Study of the Longer-Range Future.

———. 1998. *Remaking Eden*. New York: Avon.

Silvers, Anita. 1995. "Reconciling Equality to Difference: Caring (F)or Justice for People with Disabilities." *Hypatia* 10: 30–55.

———. 2000. "Super Villainous or Mild Mannered? Does Singer's Position Threaten Real People or Only Philosophically Constructed Ones?" *APA Newsletter on Philosophy and Medicine* 99, No. 2 (Spring).

———. 2009. "No Talent? Beyond the Worst Off! A Diverse Theory of Justice for Disability." In *Disability and Disadvantage*, edited by Kimberley Brownlee and Adam Cureton, 163–198. Oxford: Oxford University Press.

Silvers, Anita and Leslie Pickering Francis. 2005. "Justice Through Trust: Disability and the 'Outlier Problem' in Social Contract Theory." *Ethics* 116: 40–76.

Singer, Peter. 2000a. "Justifying Voluntary Euthanasia." In *Writings on an Ethical Life*, 194–200. New York: HarperCollins.

———. 2000b. "Severe Impairment and the Beginning of Life." *APA Newsletter on Philosophy and Medicine* 99, No. 2 (Spring).

———. 2010. "Speciesism and Moral Status." In *Cognitive Disability and Its Challenge to Moral Philosophy*, edited by Eva Feder Kittay and Licia Carlson, 331–344. Wiley-Blackwell.

———. 2011. "Parental Choice and Human Improvement." In *Human Enhancement*, edited by Julian Savulescu and Nick Bostrom. Oxford, UK: Oxford University Press.

Smit, Chris. 2013. "The Things of Disability: A Technological Phenomenology." Presentation at the Society for Disability Studies annual meeting, Orlando, FL, July 27.

Smith, Andrea. 2005. *Conquest: Sexual Violence and the American Indian Genocide*. South End Press.

Smith, Dylan, George Loewenstein, Christopher Jepson, Aleksandra Jankovich, Harold Feldman, and Peter Ubel. 2008. "Mispredicting and Misremembering: Patients with Renal Failure Overestimate Improvements in Quality of Life After a Kidney Transplant." *Health Psychology* 27, No. 5: 653–658.

Smith, S.E. 2013. "Yet Another Disabled Child Killed By Family." *XO Jane* June 19. Accessed June 15, 2014: http://www.xojane.com.

Smith, Steven R. 2009. "Social Justice and Disability: Competing Interpretations of the Medical and Social Models." In *Arguing about Disability: Philosophical Perspectives*. edited by Kristjana Kristiansen, Simo Vehmas, and Tom Shakespeare, 15–29. New York: Routledge.

Snyder, Sharon L. and David T. Mitchell. 2006. *Cultural Locations of Disability*. Chicago: University of Chicago Press.

Sober, Eliott. 2000. "The Meaning of Genetic Causation." In *From Chance to Choice: Genetics and Justice*, edited by Allen Buchanan, Daniel Brock, Norman Daniels, and Daniel Wikler, 347–370. Cambridge: Cambridge University Press.

Sontag, Susan. 1978/1989. *Illness as Metaphor and AIDS and its Metaphors*. New York: Anchor Books, Doubleday.

Sparrow, Robert. 2008. "Genes, Identity, and the 'Expressivist' Critique." In *The Sorting Society: The Ethics of Genetic Screening and Therapy*, edited by Janna Thompson and Loane Skene, 111–132. Cambridge: Cambridge University Press.

———. 2011. "A Not-So-New Eugenics: Harris and Savulescu on Human Enhancement." *The Hastings Center Report* (January-February): 32–42.

Spelman, Elizabeth V. 2002. "'Race' and the Labor of Identity." In *The Subject of Care Feminist Perspectives on Dependency*, edited by Eva Feder Kittay and Ellen K. Feder, 334–347. New York: Rowman & Littlefield.

Stark, Cynthia A. 2007. "How to Include the Severely Disabled in a Contractarian Theory of Justice." *The Journal of Political Philosophy* 15: 127–145.

Steinbock, Bonnie. 2000. "Disability, Prenatal Testing, and Selective Abortion." In *Prenatal Testing and Disability Rights*, edited by Erik Parens and Adrienne Asch, 108–123. Washington, DC: Georgetown University Press.

Stevenson, Jennifer L., Bev Harp, and Morton Ann Gernsbacher. 2011. "Infantilizing Autism." *Disability Studies Quarterly* 31, No. 3.

Stiker, Henri-Jacques. 1999. *A History of Disability*. Ann Arbor: University of Michigan Press.

Stock, Gregory. 1993. *Metaman: The Merging of Humans and Machines into a Global Superorganism*. New York: Simon and Schuster.

———. 2002. *Redesigning Humans: Our Inevitable Genetic Future*. Boston: Houghton Mifflin Harcourt.

Thompson, Larry. 1989. "The Price of Knowledge: Genetic Tests that Predict Dire Conditions Become a Two-Edged Sword." *The Washington Post* October 10.

Titchkosky, Tanya. 2002. "Cultural Maps: Which Way to Disability?" In *Disability/Postmodernity: Embodying Disability Theory*, edited by Mairian Corker and Tom Shakespeare, 101–111. New York: Continuum.

Tremain, Shelley. 2001. "On The Government of Disability." *Social Theory and Practice* 27, No. 4: 617–636.

———. 2002. "On the Subject of Impairment." In *Disability/Postmodernity: Embodying Political Theory*, edited by Marian Corker and Tom Shakespeare, 32–47. London: Continuum.

———. 2006. "Reproductive Freedom, Self-Regulation, and the Government of Impairment in Utero." *Hypatia* 21, No. 1: 35–53.

———. 2008. "The Biopolitics of Bioethics and Disability." *Bioethical Inquiry* 5: 101–106.

———. 2010. "Biopower, Styles of Reasoning, and What's Still Missing from the Stem Cell Debates." *Hypatia* 25, No. 3 (Summer): 577–609.

———. 2013. Review of *Why Have Children: The Ethical Debate* by Christine Overall. *APA Newsletter on Feminism and Philosophy*.

U.S. National Library of Medicine. 2013. "Handbook." In the *Genetics Home Reference* March 25. Accessed March 26. http://ghr.nlm.nih.gov/handbook/howgeneswork/epigenome.

Veerman, J. Lennart. 2011. "On the Futility of Screening for Genes That Make You Fat." *PLoS Med* 8, No. 11: e1001114. doi:10.1371/journal.pmed.1001114.

Waldschmidt, Anne. 1992. "Against Selection of Human Life—People with Disabilities Oppose Genetic Counselling." *Issues in Reproductive and Genetic Engineering* 5, No. 2: 155–167.

———. 2005. "Who Is Normal? Who Is Deviant? 'Normality' and 'Risk' in Genetic Diagnostics and Counseling." In *Foucault and the Government of Disability*, edited by Shelley Tremain, 191–207. Ann Arbor: University of Michigan Press.

Walters, Suzanna Danuta. 2014. *The Tolerance Trap: How God, Genes, and Good Intentions are Sabotaging Gay Equality*. New York: New York University Press.

Ware, Linda P. 2002. "A Moral Conversation on Disability: Risking the Personal in Educational Contexts." *Hypatia* 17, No. 3: 143–172.

Wapner, Ronald J. et al. 2012. "Chromosomal Microarray versus Karyotyping for Prenatal Diagnosis." *The New England Journal of Medicine* 367, No. 23: 2175–2184.

Wasserman, David. 2012. "Ethics of Human Enhancement and its Relevance to Disability Rights." *eLS*. Chichester: John Wiley & Sons, Ltd. doi: 10.10001/9780470015902.a0024135.

Weir, Lorna. 1996. "Recent developments in the government of pregnancy." *Economy and Society* 25, No. 3: 372–392.

———. 2006. *Pregnancy, Risk and Biopolitics: On the Threshold of the Living Subject*. New York: Routledge.

Wendell, Susan. 1996. *The Rejected Body: Feminist Philosophical Reflections on Disability*. New York: Routledge.

———. 2010. "Toward a Feminist Theory of Disability." In *The Disability Studies Reader*, edited by Lennard J. Davis, 260–278. New York: Routledge.

Wiggam, Albert. 1934. "Wanted: A 'Eugenics Conscience.'" *Physical Culture: The Personal Problem Magazine* (August): 16–18, 69–70.

Wolbring, Gregor. 2008. "The Politics of Ableism." *Development* 51: 252–258.

———. 2009. "'Therapeutic,' Enhancement Enabling, Assistive Devices and the UN Convention of the Rights of Persons with Disabilities: A Missing Lens in the Enhancement Regulation Discourse." *Journal of International Biotechnology Law* 6: 192–203.

Wolfe, Cary. 2009. *What is Posthumanism?* Minneapolis: University of Minnesota Press.

A World Without Bodies: Nazi Euthanasia Programs and the Deviant Body. 2001. DVD Directed by Sharon Snyder, Brace Yourselves Productions. 35 minutes.

Young, Simon. 2006. *Designer Evolution: A Transhumanist Manifesto*. New York: Prometheus Books.

Zola, Irving Kenneth. 1993. "Self, Identity and the Naming Question: Reflections on the Language of Disability." *Social Science and Medicine* 36, No. 2: 167–173.

Index

About the Author

Melinda C. Hall is an assistant professor of philosophy at Stetson University, where she teaches bioethics, ethics, and Continental philosophy. Much of her work deals with questions in bioethics and the philosophy of disability, and her ongoing research interests include emerging technologies, reproduction, and risk analysis. She received her Ph.D. in philosophy from Vanderbilt University. Her work is published in the *International Journal of Feminist Approaches to Bioethics*, *Philosophy Compass*, and *Disability Studies Quarterly*, among other venues.